Adrenal Fatigue

Restoring Your Hormones and Controlling Thyroidism

(Healing Your Hormones, and Transforming Your Lifestyle to Reclaim Your Health)

Anthony Jones

Published By **Bengion Cosalas**

Anthony Jones

All Rights Reserved

Adrenal Fatigue: Restoring Your Hormones and Controlling Thyroidism (Healing Your Hormones, and Transforming Your Lifestyle to Reclaim Your Health)

ISBN 978-1-77485-957-5

No part of this guidebook shall be reproduced in any form without permission in writing from the publisher except in the case of brief quotations embodied in critical articles or reviews.

Legal & Disclaimer

The information contained in this ebook is not designed to replace or take the place of any form of medicine or professional medical advice. The information in this ebook has been provided for educational & entertainment purposes only.

The information contained in this book has been compiled from sources deemed reliable, and it is accurate to the best of the Author's knowledge; however, the Author cannot guarantee its accuracy and validity and cannot be held liable for any errors or omissions. Changes are periodically made to this book. You must consult your doctor or get professional medical advice before using any of the suggested remedies, techniques, or information in this book.

Upon using the information contained in this book, you agree to hold harmless the Author from and against any damages, costs, and expenses, including any legal fees potentially resulting from the application of any of the information provided by this guide. This disclaimer applies to any damages or injury caused by the use and application, whether directly or indirectly, of any advice or information presented, whether for breach of contract, tort, negligence, personal injury, criminal intent, or under any other cause of action.

You agree to accept all risks of using the information presented inside this book. You need to consult a professional medical practitioner in order to ensure you are both able and healthy enough to participate in this program.

Table Of Contents

Chapter 1: Basic Bio 101 _____ 1

Chapter 2: Patient History _____ 13

Chapter 3: Second Opinion _____ 24

Chapter 4: Treatment _____ 41

Chapter 5: The Body's Response To Stress In A Natural Way _____ 51

Chapter 6: What Is Adrenal Deficiency? 172

Chapter 1: Basic Bio 101

To get an understanding of the full spectrum of the effects of adrenal fatigue it is crucial to determine the roles the adrenaline performs within your body. Before the advent of modern technology there was a lack of understanding of the special nature of the adrenals. The advances in the field of human biology has been advancing rapidly over the past few decades and have allowed medical science to slowly discover the secrets of the adrenal glands. Therefore, everything that is discussed in this chapter is based upon an outline of the specific area of endocrinology.

Adrenal Glands

All animals in the animal world have adrenal glands including powerful single-cell organisms. It's only natural that humans also have these essential organs. The adrenal glands comprise a set of triangular-shaped organs which create key hormones that allow the internal organs to function properly.

It is vital to take note that, prior to that fifteenth Century Italian biologist Bartolomeo Esutachi, humanity has no understanding of the adrenaline glands. Esutachi was among the few scientists to be credited with the development the human anatomy field as a crucial field of biology. Apart from renal function, Bartolomeo Eustachi is also recognized as the pioneer of the first detailed study of the anatomy of vital organs, such as the heart, the ear as well as the brain and the spinal cord.

The word adrenaline originates from the combination of two Latin terminologies. Ad is a word that means "near" while the term"renes" translates to "kidneys". This is the most likely explanation for their exact position in the human body. They are situated above the two organs that are responsible for removing waste residues in the circulatory system.

Each adrenaline gland have a measurement standard three inches of length, as well as 1.5 inches high. If we have to draw a comparative layman comparison the adrenaline glands are similar to the size of an acorn, or walnut, in the size of its average. The adrenaline glands weigh approximately 4 grams. In terms of appearance each of the glands look quite different in comparison to one another. Its left side appears like a curving mass looking like a Cudgel, or an odd crescent. Its right side has an equidistant resemblance to the shape of a mound. Each gland is composed of two distinct parts.

The adrenal cortex forms the outside portion of the gland which creates hormones which play a crucial function in the internal organs. This part that is outside that is the adrenaline gland produces cortisol, an enzyme which regulates metabolism. Another biochemical element produced from the adrenal cortex aldosterone. It is the principal component responsible for controlling blood pressure of the body.

The adrenal medulla, also known as the gland's inner part which is responsible for the production of hormonal substances that have been classified as not essential. It is surprising, however, that the primary hormones released from the adrenaline gland's interior are consist of the adrenaline that is named after it. According to a simplistic definition adrenaline allows the body to deal with the stressors. It is interesting to note that the adrenal medulla is only 10% of the total amount for each adrenaline gland's structures.

Anatomical Physiology

As previously mentioned The primary function of the adrenaline glands is to regulate the body's functioning and allow it to manage stress. It is essential to think about the reality that each function is interdependent with each other. That is, the body can't maintain its normal functioning when it is not able to handle anxiety. In the same way, it is impossible for the body to over come trauma if its organs and tissues are in poor condition.

The fact that this is settled, it's time to look into a more crucial question regarding the adrenal glands: What exactly is the adrenaline glands function?

The adrenaline glands are responsible for our body's "fight or reaction to flight". It is essential to understand the nature of the human body. It is constantly under pressure from a variety of sources. The stressors can be injury, infection, or emotions that are negative, such as temper, anxiety and even sadness. Whatever the way one might be able to react when confronts a stressful situation The primary function of the adrenaline glands are to stop the body from failing completely.

As we discussed in the prior section of this book cortisol and other hormones are responsible for controlling the metabolism of the body. Also known as "stress hormones" cortisol, aldosterone and aldosterone are the two main hormones that regulate blood pressure and metabolism by triggering the following physiological functions:

They increase the body's utilization of fats and carbohydrates.

They efficiently transform proteins and fats into energy.

They help to ensure the proper distribution of stored fats.

They help regulate glucose levels in the blood.

They improve the effectiveness of the central nervous system.

They boost the body's immune response.

They enhance the body's anti-inflammatory abilities.

They boost the overall cardiovascular efficiency of the body.

They regulate the overall gastrointestinal metabolism.

These physiological adjustments allow the body to respond more efficiently when confronted by stressors. There are many kinds of increased abilities when adrenaline glands are activated. fighting or flight mechanism.

The most well appreciated examples can be best illustrated by stressful situations of confrontation. Imagine a frail, asthmatic teenager boy who is escaping or protecting oneself from a small number of school bullies. A fully functioning adrenaline glands trigger a variety of physiological reactions to prepare the body to the exact demands needed to complete a certain sequence of actions. If the victim chooses to flee, he'll be running faster and feel an increase in endurance due to an abruptly increased heart rate. If the victim chooses to defend himself, the successful utilization of energy and the distribution of nutrients throughout the body will enable him to strike more effective and precise strikes, as well as successfully avoid or block an attack from an opponent because of the increased reaction times. In either case, the innocent person turns into a fully functioning combative due to the excellent adrenaline gland.

In the particular scenario discussed in the previous paragraph tension and anxiety trigger an adrenaline system. This triggers the adrenal glands to deliver an increase in physical performance. It is crucial to note that frequency and duration of a good adrenal reaction isn't as certain than one would think. Sometimes, stress overpowers the normal fighting or flee response. If this occurs the asthmatic teenage boy is inevitably subjected to another session of physical or mental violence from his abusers.

Balance and Checks on the Adrenal System and Balance

The subchapter before found that the adrenaline mechanism might occasionally suffer from a malfunction. In taking the preceding scenario into account it is easy to blame the inability to deal tension as "one incident of bad luck". But, there's an understanding of the reason the your body's performance has decreased. The reason that adrenaline glands may not perform well when it comes to dealing the stress of life is that there is not enough or too much "stress hormones" released through the glands. It is logical that cortisol's release must meet the required quantity and duration.

These are the results that result from having excess cortisol both in terms duration and total quantity:

The body is likely to have more abdominal fat. It's logical to conclude that the increase in waistline is usually connected to health issues caused by excessive levels of bad cholesterol.

The body may suffer from hyperglycemia, more commonly referred to in the form of "sugar rush". This is why people might experience anxiety and impairment (erratic) thinking. In the end, it will end with the form of a "sugar crash" and the person may experience fatigue and intense fatigue.

The body may experience increase in blood pressure, with the patient to feel lightheaded at best or migraine and vertigo at the extreme.

The body will experience a diminished muscles weight (muscle atrophy). In turn, individuals are more to be at risk of developing cardiovascular ailments due to excessive fats. The fact is that the composition of the muscles can be a major aspect of an individual's overall health. In addition, a lack of muscle mass leads in the slow healing of the open injury.

The body will show an eroding bone density. In addition to the obvious lack of energy caused by this condition An individual is at an increased risk of suffering from bone fractures due to a small blunt injury.

Additionally, the results of having a low level of cortisol are as follows:

The body can feel tired especially during the hours in the morning when your energy levels are at their highest (e.g. early morning or midday).

The body may suffer from hypoglycemia. The imbalance in glucose can cause a person to be unwell, irritable and depressed. The symptoms are similar to the symptoms of a wide range of mild symptoms of starvation.

The body is likely to have reduced blood pressure. Similar to hypertension, low blood pressure is a cause of nausea, lightheadedness and a collapse due to exhaustion in the most.

The body can suffer from inflammation. This means that a person has a higher chance to suffer the appearance of skin lesions or swelling because of mild allergies and other triggers of the immune system.

The bottom line is that both ends of the spectrum affects the various aspects of life:

Sleep quality

Understanding level

Immunity levels to infections

Chapter 2: Patient History

The previous chapter covered several important points to think about when understanding the structure and functions of adrenaline glands. In addition to its discovery within the early 15th Century the adrenaline glands were not ever known about them up to in the 21st Century. Modern medicine has revealed that the adrenaline glands have been deemed to be the origin of a biochemical mechanism to cope to combat stress. Like other important organs the adrenaline glands are in turn, at best, susceptible to malfunction, and at worst, complete failure.

The book's first chapter is dedicated to understanding the fundamentals that help explain why the adrenaline glands are ineffective. The chapter on adrenaline glands you'll not only learn about the history and causes of fatigue in adrenal glands as condition in medical science. It will also help you determine if "your" adrenal glands are in poor state. Take note that the information you gather about symptoms is only an overview. Always, it's recommended to undergo a medical evaluation to determine the assurance of one's physical health.

Chronology

Addison's Disease

The first study that was substantiated about the adrenaline glands' failure can be traced back to the 1800's. In the 19th Century English doctor Dr. Thomas Addison presented his revolutionary medical research to the South London Medical Society in 1849. According to his dissertation his findings on the "general condition of anemia that is common to males who were adults" suggested the weak adrenaline glands as the cause of similar symptoms seen in a variety of cases (e.g. lack of energy as well as a weak immune system etc.). Since then, this impairment was known as Addison's Disease, courtesy of its inventor.

Swine Serum

After the Dr. Addison's discovery of known endocrinal illness, doctors have devoted considerable effort in finding out the cause and cure for this disease. But the first important treatment method was not discovered until the year 1898. The Canadian doctor (and one of two pioneers of modern medical practice's "residency program) called Sir William Osler created a treatment for Addison's Disease using the adrenal cells of an animal. It is crucial to take note that, despite numerous successes of Dr. Osler's attempts to advance modern medical practices to the highest levels, his treatment with pigs was a dead point. Thankfully, the next generation of doctors will develop a better adrenal extract system to treat patients.

The Schism

New developments in understanding this area of endocrinology has led to some discord among medical professionals during the 20th century. As time passes during the latest waves of medical research the divergence of the consensus of all doctors becomes more apparent. Some medical professionals have been instrumental in the development of the condition known as hypoadrenia which is a term that dates back to the past for adrenal fatigue.

In 1919 in 1919, in 1919, an Italian medical professor known as Nicola Pende has clarified what hypoadrenia actually is. According to Pende, the illness is defined by an imbalance in hormones, which is often linked to benign or latent disorders of the glands that regulate the endocrine system. This, in addition to other reasons, was resisted by those who believe that it is merely a visible (physical) problem exists in the endocrine glands overall.

Accreditation Failure

Since the beginning of 1900 the diagnosis of hypoadrenia has become difficult. Because there isn't a test that can precisely diagnose an apparent mild or latent adrenal defects the analysis is dismissed as insignificant. If there's something that is difficult in the field of medical practice, it's the issue of uncertainty. From the 1920's until 1940's the medical opinions that were not certified by a medical professional concerning adrenal fatigue have not made it into the canon of medical practice. Also, all forms of treatment were treated with equally skeptical views (if not outright rejection). It could take a long period of time before a lot of attention is paid to this particular topic.

Renegade Doctors

Hypoadrenia and adrenal fatigue didn't experience an improvement until the 90's. At this point a American doctor known as Dr. James Wilson has found the method to assess symptoms of fatigue in the adrenal gland with a significant amount of accuracy. A very powerful methods that are a part of Dr. Wilson's research is saliva cortisol test. Other doctors who contributed to the understanding the issue of fatigued adrenals in modern medical practice include the Dr. Richard Shames,

Dr. Christiane Northrup and Dr. Michael Lam.

Unfortunately, despite the effort of reputable doctors such as Dr. Wilson, there still is a strong resistance to adrenal fatigue being a definitive medical diagnosis. It is among the many instances in which the majority of the medical community in general is not sure despite the increasing popularity and acceptance by the general society.

Survey Quiz

In addition to inventing"adrenal fatigue" as a term "adrenal fatigue" James Wilson, Dr. James Wilson has also created a way for non-physicians to have a decent diagnosis of a medical health. Burnout Questionnaire Burnout Questionnaire is aimed at giving an average evaluation that will determine "whether or not you're experiencing adrenal fatigue". It is important to note that regardless of the conclusion drawn from the results of the test It is recommended to seek a medical advice to identify the specific illness and the severity of the problem and the best procedure to treat the issue.

Here's this list of the questions each one to be scored from between 0 and five (with 5 , being considered the highest amount) according to intensity

Do you get tired more easily?

Do you feel tired more than you feel energetic?

Are you annoyed when people tell youthat "you aren't looking as good lately"?

Are you putting in more effort but getting less done?

Are you becoming more cynical and angry?

Do you experience a lot of unanswered grief?

Do you find yourself frequently forgetting deadlines, appointments, or other personal items?

Are you getting more sensitive?

Are you more ill-tempered?

Are you unhappy with your surroundings?

Are you seeing close family members and friends less often?

Is completing a regular task (e.g. writing reports, sending brief cards to your friends, or taking important phone calls) too much within your timetable?

Do you notice an increase in the number of physical symptoms (e.g. joint or muscle pains headaches, chronic flu or colds, etc.)?

Are you feeling disoriented after your day's activities stop?

Does happiness seem to be a elusive concept or an experience?

Are you not able to smile or make fun of you?

Sex seems like an uneasy act rather than a pleasure?

Do you have nothing to say to others?

After entering the numbers for each question, you will need to determine the average score ("total amount" subtracted in "the the total amount of questions"). The result will be used to determine your rough diagnose. Interpretation of results can be according to:

From 0 -25: the individual performing well.

26-35 The stress of the person is beginning to show.

36 - 50 This person may be a candidate for burnout

Between 51 and 65 This person is burnt out

Over 65: A person is at risk of becoming exhausted

The disease is known as adrenal fatigue, there's an excellent reason that it is that Dr. Wilson used exhaustion as an important relationship. In addition to the obvious meaning that the word "compound noun" implies "adrenal fatigue" debility (e.g. psychological, emotional, and physical) practically covers every possible medical diagnosis of the human health condition. However Burnout Questionnaire is a preliminary level of analysis. Burnout Questionnaire only provides a initial level of analysis.

The signs

It's not just was covered in the two earlier chapters. In the sense that detractors are concerned, the adrenal fatigue is an untrue disease. Many have cited its wide (and possible non-conclusive) manifestations as the root of the ambiguous diagnosis for adrenal fatigue. What are the real symptoms of this uncertain disease?

Before diving into that you must take into consideration that adrenal fatigue is a condition that can be explained by a certain basic scientific theory. Based on the Dr. Wilson; physical, emotional, and mental exhaustion may be caused by the inability of the adrenaline glands produce the proper quantity of cortisol. Based on this premise adrenal fatigue is justifiable by the following physical signs:

Symptom #1.

It's difficult to get up.

Symptom #2.

Tiredness that is constant even after getting up in the early morning.

Symptom #3.

Problems with thinking straight or finishing an assignment.

These are only the first symptoms that could develop into something more serious. Like other degenerative illnesses such as cancer and Alzheimer's Disease, adrenal fatigue may progress into a more severe version of the initial diagnosis. Additional information on Stages of Adrenal Fatigue will be covered in Chapter 3 of the book.

Chapter 3: Second Opinion

The earlier parts of the book focused on the nature of the adrenaline glands as well as the stress hormones that they produce and also an introduction to the adrenal glands as a disorder. As we discussed in the prior chapter the adrenal fatigue condition is a difficult disease to define. There's more to the unrelenting doubt of critics regarding the problem of the diagnosis of hypoadrenia. In this chapter you'll be able to draw a line and come to your own conclusions regarding the controversies between two schools of medical belief regarding the controversy surrounding adrenal fatigue.

Faux Diagnosis

The biggest challenge in diagnosing the presence of adrenal fatigue lies in that this type of condition is akin to a range of conditions by the signs in and of itself. In the preceding chapter, the initial examination is restricted to three major indicators. A chronic fatigue or lack of focus and inability to get out of the bed are essentially an ineffective set of criteria , which, by themselves can't offer an accurate analysis without continuing levels of physical analysis (e.g. reviewing the patient's information, cortisol laboratory test and thorough observation).

Ruling Out: Level One

The three mentioned specific symptoms of fatigue may be present in different, but not related conditions. These conditions include anemia, arthritis and thyroid issues, diabetes and heart disease. However, concluding that they are other ailments could be a bit premature. In reality, exhaustion may be a normal part of itself without any other underlying condition. It could manifest as a body's natural response to unhealthy lifestyles:

Poor diet

Sleeping patterns that aren't optimal

Insufficient stress management and poor the balance of work and life

Psychological depression

These are only the instances of possible conclusion that has nothing to do with relate to the body's endocrine system. In the meantime, the physician is already able to identify the cause of physical exhaustion due to other factors that are not related. What happens if the initial tests (if performed correctly) indicate a problem in the adrenaline glands that is manifested through the insufficient hormone cortisol production? Did the doctor already find the mysterious adrenal fatigue? But not so fast...

Ruling Out: Level Two

The previous chapter discussed the way in which medical professionals are split in the controversy over adrenal fatigue. As compared to adrenal fatigue Addison's Disease is an easier condition to identify since it is easy to identify in medical tests that are specific to the case. It is essentially, Addison's Disease is a problem with the adrenal glands that result from a weak immune system. It is interesting to note that this condition can be a byproduct or a symptom of another non-endocrine deficiencies. The following are serious conditions that cause Addison's Disease.

Cancer (e.g. lymphoma)

Advanced Immune Deficiency Syndrome (AIDS)

Tuberculosis

Be aware: Addison's Disease is concluded through the examination of the damage done to the adrenal glands. One or both of the adrenaline glands expand or shrink, suffer minor lesions or suffer from some other visible deformities. The major difference between the condition with adrenal fatigue and the former is "the adrenal fatigue's lack of cortisol is not due to any physical or chemical damage". Incredibly, Addison's Disease is not only just a result of the three most common signs of physical, mental or emotional fatigue. In addition to general fatigue, there are other symptoms that indicate the need to diagnose Addison's Disease:

Darkening pigmentation on the joints and palms

The feeling of dizziness when standing up

Menstrual cycle is not a regular part of the routine for females

A condition like adrenal fatigue is susceptible to being a false diagnosis as a result of the numerous factors that doctors must determine. It is normal for a lot of doctors to think that the detection of adrenal fatigue is simply something that is a "wild hunt" and not worthy of serious focus. In the medieval era the apothecaries would have reached the same conclusion about complicated diseases like tuberculosis, because of the apparent inexperience, lack of information and resources.

Top 10 Facts

Concerning the difficulty of identifying adrenal fatigue one must consider an analogy similar to that in terms of security for the nation. So even though terrorists can be difficult to identify isn't a guarantee that they aren't there. In the world of pure science of medicine, skepticism is present as an integral part of every possible method of investigation until all possibilities of finding them exhausted.

Doctor. Michael Lam is one of the main advocates of adrenal fatigue in the mid 1990's. Although his colleague Dr. James Wilson, described the nature of the controversial condition, Dr. Michael Lam has laid out ten easy facts to dispel the widespread doubts about adrenal fatigue. Below are "progressive" explanations that justify the validity that adrenal fatigue is a real issue:

1. The real cause of fatigue is adrenal fatigue.

The most efficient method for the proof of a particular concept or idea is affirming that it is valid. One method is to give a clear definition. According Dr. Lam, adrenal fatigue is a health issue that can be traced to a variety of symptoms that are not specific to.

2. The signs of fatigued adrenal glands are numerous and diverse.

In addition to the general exhaustion, there are numerous symptoms to be considered. They include anxiety, insomnia and low blood pressure muscles pain, etc. In the end, "oversimplification" is not always the most effective way to tackle a complicated issue.

3. Our understanding of the adrenal fatigue phenomenon is still in the early stages.

Like many shrewd scientists Lam, like many of the most eminent scientists. Lam recognizes the current limitations of medical technology of the present. Through analogy the inability to locate an armed terrorist doesn't mean that they don't exist. It's arrogance to believe that there's no space for improvement in the field of medical research.

4. A lot of the signs of adrenal fatigue can be attributed to hormones.

Because symptoms of adrenal fatigue are related to hormones, traditional forms treatments are intended to alleviate the initial discomfort. But, merely reducing symptoms can mask the root cause of hormonal imbalance. Therefore, traditional methods of treatment are often a shortsighted approach which is likely to not work in the long run.

5. Every person's biochemical nature is different for each person.

A second inviolable truth the Dr. Lam seeks to impart is the intricate nature of individual physiological processes. In this regard, it's almost impossible to make a diagnosis from a variety of responses from patients. Some patients might exhibit severe symptoms that are not related to adrenal fatigue while some might suffer from adrenal fatigue, but not show any indications.

6. Adrenal fatigue is real and painful.

Adrenalin fatigue crashes are common when you have exhausted the immediate response to stress-related conditions. The reason for this is the body's inability of recovering quickly from the resulting reactions. In the most severe instances patients may become sick after just being in a stressful situation. The body returns to its normal levels of energy to "feel secure".

7. A proper nutritional supplementation is essential to help recover.

Through the term "proper" By the adjective "proper," Dr. Lam suggests that consumption of nutritional supplements needs to be carefully monitored regarding dose and frequency. The reason that recommended treatments fail is due to the fact that patients aren't under constant supervision regarding the administration of the treatment.

8. Exercise can aid in the recovery of your adrenal gland however, it must be done in a way that is safe.

Alongside nutritional supplements, a different corrective procedure that is under strict supervision is exercising. According Dr. Lam, a patient should not exert too much, or it can cause adrenal fatigue and crash. In the end, a great exercise shouldn't cause pressure or stress. The most important thing is that a successful exercise must be supported by a healthy and balanced diet.

9. The standard blood test isn't very helpful.

In contrast to other chronic diseases the traditional blood test cannot be used to diagnose adrenal fatigue. Through analogy, it is possible to consider this test as a way to stereotype ethnic groups to describe a person's character. In the words of Professor Dr. Lam would put it, "a single snapshot of one's hormone function at a specific time point rarely is all that accurate and actually, it could be deceiving.

10. The secret to complete recovery from adrenal fatigue is getting a skilled professional.

According to Dr. Lam is concerned, the most effective method to combat the issue of adrenal fatigue (given the present stage of infancy when it comes to knowing the cause of this condition) is to take an integrative "mind-body" method. This involves a mix of lifestyle modifications, diet along with nutritional supplements. A more detailed explanation of the overall treatment will be provided in Chapter 4 in this book.

The stages of illness

It is more than just a definition and a clear set of evidence to determine the authenticity of a particular disease. Adrenal fatigue advocates didn't just conclude that this condition is real enough to be dismissed They have also claimed that adrenal fatigue requires the most attention.

Similar to other serious chronic diseases (e.g. AIDS tuberculosis cancer) adrenal fatigue too is a chronic condition that is classified into different stages. Here's the essential outline of each stage from the joint research of adrenal fatigue sufferers:

Phase 1: Alarm Phase

The initial phase of adrenal fatigue can be marked by mild signs of exhaustion. Due to the difficulty of making an exact diagnosis at this phase and the presence of the alarm, it often doesn't even show the obvious signs that are mentioned in the last two chapters in this book. In the end, the adrenal glands are functioning normally in the sense that they are capable of producing an enormous quantity of hormones to keep with the stressors.

However, laboratory tests could indicate a slight rise in levels of cortisol, epinephrineand androstenolone steroid (DHEA) and insulin. The basic idea is that a person might experience a lot of exuberance and alertness. Therefore, a person may be somewhat more anxious than regular people. In direct consequence of these bursts of energy, an individual could experience irregular sleeping patterns as well as alternating fatigue.

Stage 2: The Continuing Phase

At this point it is possible that a more obvious hormonal imbalance could be observed. Although the endocrine system is capable of responding to stressors, the usual amount of sex hormones could start to diminish. In reality the adrenaline glands are not able to multitask between helping the body manage stress and also producing hormones that regulate sexual desire. When it comes to the body's health is concerned, the need for self-defense is more important. These organs produce more stress hormones but fewer sexual hormones.

As a result of the amount of hormonal imbalance someone who is suffering from stage 2 adrenal fatigue might be "wired but exhausted". In exchange for increased levels of consciousness in the day the person might experience an extended exhaustion in the evening when the body's energy drops in the evening. One particular sign can be related to a high dependency of stimulants (e.g. chocolate bars or coffee) to help sustain oneself for the remainder of the waking hours. In this phase one may not always require a visit to the doctor, however certain patterns might receive the full focus.

Third Stage: Phase of Resistance

As the body enters that Resistance Phase, the ability of the adrenal glands to create testosterone and other hormones for sexual pleasure is "totally" assigned to the production of stress hormones. The ability to make the natural hormones and testosterone (among other things) is delayed in order to adapt to cortisol production "hectic" cortisol levels.

A person may be able to maintain a normal life (e.g. maintain an occupation, maintain friendships with friends, or even complete basic chores). But, living quality starts to decline because of a lack of passion. It requires a lot of effort to get sexually excited and, at worst romances might start to exhibit indications of being strained. Physically, the sufferer is often exhausted and may be more susceptible to certain illnesses (e.g. the seasonal influenza).

The physical discomforts can be more difficult to deal with since they happen over in longer intervals, some lasting months to heal while others are suffering for many years to be. Stage 3 is the most prominent juncture in the various stages that are associated with adrenal fatigue. It is often at this stage that patients would be prompted to seek consultation with their doctors.

Stage 4: Phase of Burnout

The state of adrenal fatigue has made the person a complete unstable. In the burnout Phase the body's ability to make stress as well as sexual hormones is in a gradual diminution. The body is losing base in the fight against stress.

A person who is suffering from stage 4 adrenal fatigue has already been afflicted by fatigue and extreme exhaustion. Other physical issues are sudden weight loss as well as more frequent and long-lasting infections. Sometimes, people can also experience a deterioration in memory. It is a lot of effort to concentrate on a simple task, and it becomes difficult to complete tasks done. This is why job performance can become extremely poor and one could be in danger of losing their job.

Sexually stimulating experiences were an unrecollection of a younger. Psychologically speaking, someone experiencing this stage of adrenal fatigue also experiencing a higher rate of antisocial episodes. They are most likely to stay away from social interactions and is often annoyed. The person who is at this point tends to be depressed, apathetic and cynical. They are overtaken by negative feelings. In the worst case you may think that life is meaningless.

It is crucial for people who are experiencing level 4 of adrenal fatigue, to get help immediately by a qualified medical professional. The treatment is a total lifestyle change. Similar to hypertension and other chronic diseases it is almost impossible to reverse completely the damage caused by the Burnout Phase within the given time frame. The possibility exists to overcome this condition, but it needs to be treated even after initial symptoms have decreased. Treatment requires a long-term commitment as severe symptoms could recur as the patient "takes their step off of the accelerator".

Chapter 4: Treatment

In the previous two chapters The adrenal fatigue condition is pretty extremely a numbing condition. What makes it particularly ominous is the fact that it is a symptom of a weakened immune system. As the Dr. Lam would put it our understanding of the condition is still in its early stages. Medical science has only begun to scratch the surface of a comprehensive understanding of adrenal fatigue. This lack of information is the most troubling factor in the treatment of this disease. The fact that there's no consensus among all members of the medical profession regarding the validity that adrenal fatigue is a condition just shows the ugliest degree of insecurity.

However an approach that is holistic to healthy living has frequently stood up to scrutiny for centuries regarding its effective way to fight off illness whether real or imagined. The enduring phrase "prevention is more effective than treatment" could not be more appropriate in the context of tackling the mystery of a condition such as adrenal fatigue. Through the lens of analogy, you should ask you... Do you be interested in knowing the character of a possible attacker within the dark alley rather than just staying away from the zone?

Diet Restriction

Hippocrates Hippocrates, the Ancient Greek doctor, and the founder of Western medicine, cited the most important advice that is widely followed by the modern standards of health care to this day. He wrote, "Let your food be your medicine and your medicine be your food." Since the time of the Classical Antiquities, the first step to a responsible treatment is selecting a healthy diet. The well-known 21st Century stress syndrome called adrenal fatigue is not an exempted from this ancient and inviolable norm.

Consuming the foods that are prescribed is just as crucial as keeping away from the foods that are not recommended. The shortest route to selecting your diet plan is the four keywords that are hyphenated that are nutrient-rich, high in fiber, low in sugar and cholesterol.

In order to help you create an easier diet plan we will highlight the kinds of substances that one should stay clear of. These are the food and drinks that are blacklisted by experts in adrenal fatigue:

Caffeine

It is not recommended to drink coffee for those who have suffered with adrenal fatigue. The stimulants can disrupt sleep patterns and create tension, which disrupts the capacity of adrenaline glands to heal from cortisol's excessive release. If you must drink caffeinated drinks and are consumed, they should be done so in moderation during the day.

Sugar and artificial sweeteners

Sugar consumption is a cause of numerous ailments, including hypertension and diabetes. The same principles apply to the management of adrenal fatigue since the presence of hyperglycemia can disrupt the balance of cortisol and the other stress hormones. Stevia and raw honey are the best options for giving sweetness to food.

Processed and Microwaved Foods

The primary reason microwaved and processed foods aren't recommended to people who are suspected of having adrenal fatigue has to have to do with digestion. Foods with preservatives and fillers consume a larger amount of energy to digest. In the case of dealing with adrenal fatigue the person should be able optimize their energy levels and not decrease it. It is best to consume whole meat sources such as turkey, chicken and fish that are fatty for an excellent source of minerals and protein. Nuts, seeds as well as legumes are important too.

Hydrogenated Oils

Anyone suffering from adrenal fatigue should also stay away from vegetable oils. Inflammatory substances such as hydrogenated oils can cause adrenal inflammation. The most suitable alternatives for those who consume a high fat diet is coconut oil, olive oil organic butter, and coconut oil.

Supplements

In general eating the right foods can help sustain an enduring and durable body. Unfortunately, decades of poor agricultural practices have created an environment that has compromised the quality of both crops and livestock. Vegetables are grown on synthetic media, even if they are there is no contamination of the soil. Animals on farms rely on forage that is not up to par. Therefore, the best sources of nutrients might not be sufficient to meet the requirements of a body that is suffering from adrenal fatigue.

To address this, nutritional supplements were created to help with a range different nutritional deficiencies. The following supplements will help you manage your adrenal fatigue:

* Vitamin C

* Vitamin B5

* Vitamin B12

* Vitamin D3

* Magnesium

* Zinc

* DHA (Fish oils)

* Holy basil

* Indian ginseng

Lifestyle Changes

There's more to wellness than what we consume in their bodies. Actually, the practices, personal habits and the environment play an crucial role in ensuring health. If people of ordinary age are expected to maintain a healthy lifestyle and have a healthy environment, more focus is placed on improving the general health of those who suffer from adrenal fatigue. It is logical to conclude that stress can be an essential component of our lives. The best way to manage stress is reduce your exposure to stress-related situations.

Relieve yourself when you're tired to the max.

Be aware of your body. The feeling of fatigue is a natural manifestation of the body's desire for energy replenishment. One must recognize that refusing to take a break during periods of exhaustion is an unconscious way of committing self-harm. Many people avoid the benefits of rest due to often misinterpreted ethical principles in the workplace (e.g. "a efficient person can be described as an undertaxed machine").

Keep 8-10 hours of rest each day.

The body needs at least between 8 and 10 hours rest each day. But knowing the precise time to go to bed is far more important than just sleeping for the time period that is prescribed. Do not stay awake late during a normal sleeping schedule to not strain your energy levels.

Eat at the right moment and frequency, as well as the right quantity.

In addition to the advice previously given to eat a balanced food, it's important to keep track of the time at which one chooses to consume food. For instance, a 12 hour gap between the breakfast meal and following meal is a bad eating habit that can lead to overeating and defeat the goal of the healthy diet program. When you eat at the right time, it can result in an positive domino effect. So, there's no need to increase your substance intake due to eating in a time that is too early or late than what is planned.

You can exercise at your individual pace.

Even though overexertion could harm those who are suspected of suffering from an adrenal exhaustion, inactivity can result in a deficiency production of stress hormones in a stalemate. A steady exercise routine will permit every vital organ to slowly improve (considering that there's no any underlying injury that is not resolved). Pay attention to your body and mind. If an exercise (regardless of the level of effort) does not "triggers an appropriate reward system" then it's time to put it down. There's nothing worse than exercising and feeling awful by pushing yourself until the point of breaking. There is a big distinction between working out and being exhausted.

Always try to find the positive side of your life.

In the instance of adrenal fatigue the phrase "laughter can be the most effective treatment" is just too true to be a cliché. If a person is filled with positive energy that are positive, they have greater chance of keeping and maximizing the energy. This, in essence, is a less requirement for the adrenaline glands generate stress hormones. Positive energy can reduce the possibility of exposing the person to stress.

Find counseling or help for those who are struggling.

Given that a substantial majority of those who advocate for it in the medical and lay communities have recognized adrenal fatigue to be a severe condition It is logical that no one should be forced to battle this disease on their own. The individual can only do the most with his or her own determination, efforts and determination. However, the likelihood of success can be increased by having a strong support system. The presence of people who support your growth gives you one thing that anyone can never achieve by themselves - an incentive to live.

Chapter 5: The Body's Response To Stress In A Natural Way

Stress is a body reaction to events or threats that could be detrimental to the body. If you sensed a danger like a stranger walking towards you in the dark, or a lion who roared towards you, the small area of your brain called the hypothalamus activated an alarm inside your body. This alarm is directed at addressing the danger of running for safe (fight or flight or the freeze reaction).

The prefrontal cortex and the hypothalamus assist the brain in interpreting the threat. Further processing is required to determine if the threat is real. The prefrontal cortex and hypothalamus are responsible for processing contextual events.

A lion's sight advancing towards a hunter bizarre can trigger a terror response. This triggers the hypothalamus to trigger an alarm that signals the animal to run or fight. However, the reaction to seeing the same lion inside an enclosure or in a zoo more of curiosity and demands an emotional response similar to excitement.

An event that is stressful or threatening causes the adrenal gland to release different hormones, such as cortisol and adrenaline. Adrenaline as well as noradrenaline (a similar neurotransmitter and hormone) get released in the bloodstream thereby increasing the heart and blood pressure, and providing energy to combat the threat that is perceived.

Cortisol hormones which are the main stress hormones, boost glucose or sugar levels in the bloodstream. They also enhance the glucose intake of the brain, along with increased muscular and respiratory tension and restrain body functions like reproduction and digestion, which aren't required during the stress.

It is crucial to remember that cortisol has different functions within the body, apart from the regulation of stress. It is commonly referred to as stress hormones due to their direct link in the body's stress response. The majority of cells in the body are able to respond to cortisol since it is one of the hormones that steroidize.

The psychological and physiological effect from the battle, flight or the freeze response

The hypothalamus acts as the Kickstarter telling that the adrenal gland releases cortisol and adrenaline hormones in any situation that demands the emergency response(threat).

The hormones cortisol and adrenaline increased the heart rate and directed blood flow to areas that require rapid actions.

They were first identified as early as the 1920s, by American physiological scientist Walter Cannon. Walter described the 'fight flight or freeze' reaction as a decision that people take in the face of a threat. It is either to combat and neutralize the threat, or to flee to a safer setting.

An knowledge of the "fight or run response can help you manage stress in stressful situations. Stress that is acute or daily can help us complete the tasks we have to do every day successfully. The 'fight or flight' scenario prepares our body to accomplish the job at hand.

The body's responds to stress by self-adjusting. When a threat is perceived to have been eliminated, the levels of levels of adrenaline as well as Cortisol (Stress Hormone) is restored to normal. As cortisol and adrenaline decrease the blood pressure and heart rate are restored to normal levels, and the other body systems return to normal activities. The constant threat to the body caused the 'fight or flee response to remain on.

The well-coordinated chain response triggered by the 'fight, flee or freeze' response can have both psychological and physiological impacts on the body.

A rise in blood flow can increase the supply of energy and oxygen to the lungs and heart. However you will find more glucose in your brain and skeletal muscles and enhanced eyesight improves the visual acuity to allow for better understanding of the surrounding.

Fight, fight or freeze reaction begins at the brain's amygdala (the portion of our brain that is responsible for fear, excitement and mode.

The amygdala is responsible for sending messages to the hypothalamus that controls an autonomous system of nerves. The independent nervous system is comprised of the parasympathetic system and the sympathetic system. The formal triggers an instinctive fight-or-flight reaction, while the parasympathetic system controls the freezing. Frozen is fight or flight as well as hold. It is a stoic state of dormancy, that prepares for you to defend yourself.

Fighting, fleeing or freeze reaction is a response to danger and fear. It also has physical effects on the body. The way people react to stress is different depending on their experience. A person who has survived an airplane crash may feel anxious upon seeing an aircraft. Car crash survivors might be stressed due to the car that is passing by.

The body's fight or freeze response is a psychological condition that causes fear. Trauma victims typically develop an exaggerated reaction to the perceived threat which is not the true threat.

The multiplication effect of chronic stress on the other areas within the body.

Stress caused by the constant threat of long-term, multiple stressful events could result in a prolonged drain in the physical.

The constant activation of the autonomic nervous system triggers an emotional response that results in wear and tear on the body. Imagine a sprinter working non-stop for twenty-four hours with not taking a single minute off. Imagine the constant release of cortisol and adrenaline hormones every second to assist the athlete carry on the race. Every event that is stressful that runs for a long time puts the same pressure on the nervous system's autonomous part which has a multiplier effect other body parts.

The blood vessel and the heart are the two major components of the cardiovascular system that are in synergy to supply oxygen and other nutrients to every part that comprise the human body. Stress that is prolonged can increase the risk of developing health issues for blood vessels and the heart. The continuous rise in heart rate, coupled with the elevated levels of cortisol, adrenaline, and cortisol could increase the chance of stroke, hypertension or heart attack.

People who suffer from breathing issues such as asthma or emphysema face difficult breathing during stress-related reactions. They breath faster to supply oxygen and nourish blood flow to the.

Acute stress triggers the reaction to the immune system to infections. These stimulations aid in avoiding infection and treat injuries. Stress over time reduces the immune system and helps to neutralize the body's defense against illnesses. The people who suffer from chronic stress are at risk of colds and flu as well as other ailments. They can even extend the healing time for wounds.

Stress causes the muscles of the body to be in constant alertness. Stress-related disorders can be triggered by it. For example migraine headaches can be caused by muscle tension that is prolonged in the head, shoulder and neck.

The effects of stress on the production of testosterone, and this can affect the sex drive. The nervous system is responsible for controlling sexual reproduction in males. It is the sympathetic component that triggers arousal and the parasympathetic portion is responsible for relaxation. The fight or flight response triggers testosterone and activates the sympathetic nerve system that is responsible for the arousal process. It releases cortisol as a the response to stress.

Cortisol is crucial in blood pressure regulation and the normal functioning of many body cells including male reproduction. Excel cortisol may alter the normal biological performance of the male reproductive system.

Stress increases the risk of developing type two diabetes. Stress hormones trigger an increase in glucose production inside the body and can increase the blood sugar level. If the body is in continuous stress, it could not be able to handle the increased glucose. This can increase the likelihood of developing the type 2 form of diabetes.

The Dr. Bruce Sherman McEwen, the official director of the The Harold Millikan and Margaret Millikan Hatch Lab of Neuroendocrinology, Rockefeller University, declared that "stress is linked to the aging process and depression, heart attack arthritis, rheumatoid and diabetes, as well as other diseases."

Dr. Sherman explained further that stress of extreme intensity had been proven as a weakening of the immune system. It can also stress the heart, and destroy memories in brain cells. The waist is where fat deposits are instead of the hips and buttocks.

What causes chronic stress? Allostatic Load.

Pacific salmon are born in freshwater. They then move to ocean waters for a several years before returning to freshwater, its homestead to spawn. As the Salmon increase their energy levels and race back to their homestead in order to reproduce the stress hormones, or cortisol levels rise which gives them the strength to battle the current. But, the constant rise in hormones impacts the digestive tract of the salmon, that shrinks, prompting the Salmon to cease eating. The immune system of the Salmon weakens and eventually dies due to fatigue and infections following the laying of eggs. All Pacific Salmon have been in the same loop. The rise in hormones that cause chronic stress can cause health issues that ultimately end their lives.

Humans are made by pressing the ability to fight or freeze which allows everything to return back to normal once the process of reducing the effect.

This autonomous system that regulates the fight and flight response or the freeze reaction is comprised of the parasympathetic and sympathetic system. The sympathetic response is responsible for the fight or flight reaction while the parasympathetic reaction triggers the freeze reaction.

Doctor. Stellar McEwen describes three kinds of stress. Acute or good stresscan be a reaction to a typical one-off event that provides a boost of energy and blood flow to the area of the body which required it to finish the task. Stress that is temporary, a reaction to daily disappointment when things don't turn out the way you expected. Stress that is toxic-a response to the constant toxic stream of pressures that eventually destroys the body.

In moderate quantities in moderate amounts, In moderate amounts. Bruce S.

McEwen believed that stress can be beneficial and the body's system is designed to handle it. However, people could be in danger in the event of several stressors that last longer than anticipated.

Alarms from vehicles blaring from various directions, the endless flow of traffic and suddenly appearing of large lion, answering calls, and writing letters aren't an option.

"Allostatic load" describes the psychological and physiological pressure of stress that is constantly imposed on the body. The concept of allostatic load comes from the word "Allostasis.'

The body's equilibrium is achieved via an instinctive fight-or-flight response and then normality is restored by the parasympathetic portion of our autonomous nerve system after any stressful event.

Doctor. McEwen and Dr. Sapolsky's work in the field of chronic stress first appeared in the journal Nature in the year 1968. Their research led to a new research field that revealed the ways that stress and related hormones affect human behavior as well as alter the brain and also neutralize the immune system's capability to fight infection.

If stress continues to be present for too long and continues to linger, when it is too long, Dr. Bruce explained that the normal protection system gets overwhelmed and causes what he described as 'Allostatic load', which disrupts the feedback system, causing damage.

The Dr. Bruce explained further that the burden of allostatic is exacerbated by unhealthy habits of people and their unique ways of reacting to stress.

"The reality is that we're living in a society that our systems aren't permitted to have a relax, and to return to the baseline." He said that "they are caused by excess calories, insufficient sleep, by the absence of exercise, or smoking, from isolation or the frenzied competitiveness."

Dr. Bruce later shields more light on Allostatic load in Neuropsychopharmacology 2000 journals. It says it is "In the case of anxiety disorder, depression as well as aggressive and hostile states, drug abuse, and post-traumatic stress disorder, Allostatic load is a result of chemical imbalances, as well as disturbances in the diurnal rhythm and, in some instances the brain's structures are atrophy."

Dr. Bruce further explains that one of the major risk factors for these ailments is the early experiences of abuse and neglect which can lead to a higher stress load and can lead to victims experiencing depression, social isolation or hostility, as well as overweight.

The Dr. Bruce explained further in his model that stress by itself isn't the issue, but the challenges that come with stress that result from the complicated interactions between the demands from the world outside and our body's capacity to deal with perceived threats.

This capacity is due to the bonds that we share with our support networks, hereditary and childhood experiences, sleep patterns as well as diet and exercise as well as the capacity to deal with multiple stressors at the same time.

Understanding the signs of adrenal fatigue

Those who had been to the hospital for a test to identify what they can't explain about health can relate with this common phrase by Their Endocrinologist......." it is all in your head."

Many people are frustrated when the Addison test did not come back positive, even though they've explained their symptoms to their doctor. Damage to the adrenal glands has been found to be above certain limits for an affirmative Addison test.

The test is negative, and they experience constant deficiency or a surge in cortisol. In a way it could be that the Endocrinologist could be correct!

Based on the research of Professor Dr. Joseph E. LeDoux who is an American Neuroscientist the amygdala, which is a cluster of cells that are located near the bottom of the brain recognizes the first indication of danger. Its autonomous nervous system comprised of the parasympathetic and sympathetic and parasympathetic systems, determines how to react and keep track of where the threat took place to prevent recurring. Thus, it could be said that if the threat is removed and the brain becomes susceptible to damage.

Studies conducted over a decade have revealed that stress-related constant pressure and eventually the rise in cortisol could affect the hippocampus, a region of the brain. This can lead to the formation of new memories, learning, and emotions.

Research has shown that stress hormones may cause the shrinking of the hippocampus's nerve cells and stop the growth of cells. These changes are associated with memory disorders.

The production of stress hormones is high in the first hour of the day, and decreases as the day advances. Chronic stress alters the regular cortisol production circle. Stress sufferers have higher cortisol levels at baseline that produce less or too much in the wrong amount at the right time.

Cortisol principal function is to release energy during times of stress job via the release of glucose into blood. When cortisol is at its highest level it is able to work in conjunction with elevated insulin levels and ultimately causes fat to be released into the abdomen. It is associated with an increased risk of developing heart disease diabetes, cancer and other chronic diseases. However, the idea of chronic stress being an underlying cause of chronic illness like cancer is debated.

The Dr. Ellisa Epel at the University of California found that cortisol and belly fat seem to coexist even in slim women.

Chronic stress has a negative effect on our immune system the lab. The researcher Dr. Glaser from Ohio State and his wife Dr. Janice found that the average wood required an average of more than nine days for healing women with Alzheimer's patients than for those who did not take care of patients with Alzheimer's.

A lack of sexual drive can be an indication that adrenal fatigue. A study from 2014 released in the Journal of Sexual Medicine by Dr. Lisa Dawn Hamilton and Dr. Cindy Meston about women's sexual health revealed that chronic stress can have a negative impact on sexual Arousal. Researchers found that high cortisol levels and the distractions that result from stress can lead to an arousal level that is lower in a stressful environment. by chronic stress, which is the most important task for the body to recover and to survive. So, the body is likely to reduce non-essential functions like the production of sex hormones.

The adrenal gland also produces sexual hormones, apart from stress hormones. The gland produces Dehydroepiandrosterone (DHEA), which comprises the estrogen- female reproductive system and testosterone- male reproductive system. When the adrenal gland begins to tired, the levels of these sexual hormones decreases. This can result in a decrease in sexual desire.

It is also crucial to remember that other medical conditions, such as high blood pressure, diabetes heart disease, diabetes, and drugs like antidepressants may cause a decrease in sexual drive.

Depression can also be a sign of adrenal fatigue , or chronic stress. Depression is an event in which a person has frequent mood changes, including a sense of pain, sadness despair and despair. Social loneliness. Rage and anger. Incapacitation and feeling of helplessness. A loss of concentration. Involuntary, usually anxious and restless.

The Dr. James L. Wilson wrote that "people experiencing adrenal fatigue that is characterized by low cortisol/DHEAS are diagnosed clinically to also experience depression, brain frogs as well as difficulty in concentrating and less rapid recall of memories." They generally feel less accommodating as they did previously and are frequently annoyed.

A decrease in stamina and frequent morning fatigue could indicate the presence of a deficient adrenal component that contributes to depression, according to Dr. James, the author of the adrenal fatigue 21st century syndrome of stress.

The prefrontal cortex, the most advanced area of the brain that is responsible for higher-order thought. This is the brain region that is the most sensitive being exposed to stress for long periods of time.

Stress causes structural changes to the brain's prefrontal dendron. The prefrontal cortex regulates the modes of thought, action, and emotions through numerous connections to another brain region.

Patricia G. Rakic, neuroscientist, discusses how the prefrontal cortex is able to store recent events, remember details from previous events and regulate emotions, behaviors and thoughts. Alan Baddeley called this "mental sketch pad."

The prefrontal cortex guards this vital function from internal and external disturbances, and is essential for completing the day-to-day tasks and removing any actions that appear to be in the wrong direction.

The prefrontal cortex depends on the proper functioning of its neuronal network as well as its neurochemical environment. Any disruption from outside could cause mental illness, such as anxiety or depression.

Chronic anxiety and stress disorders

Anxiety refers to being overly anxious or scared to the point that you are in a position to not be able to perform daily routines. Sometimes, feeling anxious and nervous is a normal aspect of life. The normal anxiety can motivate us to reach our goals , and for example, studying for an exam!

But, when these emotions become persistent, intense and excessive the condition can become a problem that requires a professional's focus. It is often evident as a panic attack or Post-traumatic Stress Disorder.

Life events that can cause extreme stress, like the loss of a loved one, loss of job or divorce, as well as accidents could cause anxiety attacks and panic attacks.

Fear and anxiety due to perceived threats are different with actual threat. An anxiety attack is a response to a threat that is imagined.

The fear of being perceived creates an imagined hostile environment which is distinguished by its suddenness as well as its debilitating and immobilizing the intensity.

The heartbeat can be heard racing to its peak as well as breathing difficulties, as well as a feeling of being ill or depressed. Anxiety may be triggered by a fear of death (imaginary threat) as well as restlessness and anxiety.

The symptoms of anxiety triggered by stress can include stomachache, muscle tension fast breathing, sweating, headache, shaking, and dizziness.

Fatigue is the exhaustion extreme resulting of physical or mental stress or an illness. A study conducted by Anna Dahlgren and fellow published in the National Library of Medicine found that high levels of stress at work were associated with sleepiness in the evening.

The study also revealed that in any week where the overall work hours increase the overall sleep time decreases. A work week with a high workload can increase sleepiness as well as work hours, which can disrupt sleep and alters the daily cortisol release.

Insufficient sleep is an indication of fatigue. Stress can disrupt the natural sleep cycle by increasing cortisol release into the bloodstream. This influences the production of sleep hormones - Melatonin, which in turn hinders the ability to sleep.

The Dr. David Borenstain, an integrative physician and the creator of Manhattan integrative medicine, says that you experience a feeling of fatigue with low energy, and you're unable to rest when you're suffering from adrenal fatigue. The majority of people depend on stimulants such as caffeine to help you get through the day, and you'll have an overwhelming desire for salt and sugar. There are times when you may experience headaches.

The adrenal gland is a result of chronic stress

The feeling of fatigue and lack of energy top the list of reasons why patients seek assistance from Doctors. But, it can be difficult to establish the diagnosis since a variety of illnesses are associated with signs of fatigue. Medical doctors look for clues through listening, studying the medical history, conducting physical examinations and a saliva test.

But, a definitive diagnosis is still elusive regardless of all the efforts in clinical. There are a variety of theories that have been put forward in order to explain the difficult medical diagnosis and alternative therapies to aid patients ease their pain.

There are theories that suggest adrenal insufficiency due to chronic stress, fatigue and thyroid dysfunction, also known as hyperthyroidism.

Dr. Lynnette Nieman, a senior investigator of the National Institute of health and director of the endocrine consult service of the National Institute of clinical health service sent a letter to the endocrine society in order to express concern over the patients' frustration.

"Our responsibility is to be active listeners and identify if there's an appropriate medical issue lurking within the symptoms. It is vital for the patient to not brush them off and claim that there's nothing such like adrenal fatigue. They are suffering from something and we should consider them serious".

The theory of adrenal fatigue explains the fact that repeated exposure to situations that trigger stress over time could deplete the adrenal glands, causing malfunction and then mass production of cortisol timing. In normal stress adrenal glands release cortisol into bloodstreams that is converted into energy to help the body face threats that are perceived.

This chain reaction, known as fight or freeze response, is marshaled through the Hypothalamus-Pituitary-Adrenal (HPA) axis.

Adrenal glands are tiny sharp triangular glands that are located in the top of both kidneys. The adrenal glands comprise two parts: the Cortex along with the Medulla that are responsible for generating different hormones to regulate metabolism in the body.

The most notable of them are stress and sex hormones. If the adrenal glands are unable to produce the hormones required for our body, it causes adrenal insufficiency, a condition called Addison disease. The adrenal gland can become malignant due to excessive hormones. In these instances it is not a formality to say the adrenal gland suffers from fatigue or adrenal fatigue.

We aren't able to precisely what will happen to us. Everyday problems, such as navigating the traffic, or someone trying to get in a line, or a door key issue and mistaking you for locked out when keys are inside could cause stress enough to put your entire body on alert.

When stress continues to last longer than anticipated and in certain instances the system responsible for the stress response may not be capable of returning to normal. The emotion can be expressed by anger, arousal or memory could be short in duration.

This condition can manifest in the negative effects on psychological health (depression as well as anxiety) as well as frequent colds and flu, due to the inability by the immune system shield the body from external threats. Thus, fatigue can be seen in a craving for sleeping incessantly and an inability to get up early to get up.

Hypothyroidism

There is a myth regarding hyperthyroidism and adrenal fatigue. While the symptoms of the two conditions are like they are similar, there is a distinct disorders that require specific treatment.

Thyroid glands that are under- or over-active exhibit similar symptoms as adrenal fatigue. Nervousness, depression, anxiety and a constant fluctuation in body temperature and fatigue.

The signs are usually difficult to differentiate from those caused by adrenal fatigue. However, it is recommended to make sure you have a clear diagnosis prior to the beginning of the treatment.

The thyroid gland is responsible for two major hormones, which are triiodothyronine(T3) as well as thyroxine(T4). It releases these hormones into bloodstreams to be transmitted to cells.

The thyroid gland measures about 2 inches long, butterfly-shaped and is located in the front of it, just beneath Adam's apple. There are two parts known as lobes. They are connected by an by an isthmus, a bridge prototype.

It is regulated through the hypothalamus-Pituitary-thyroid gland and the hypothalamus signal to the pituitary axis--demanding the thyroid gland to produce more or less triiodothyronine(T3) and thyroxine(T4).

The pituitary and the hypothalamus continuously communicate to keep a balance of T3 Hormones and T3. The hormones regulate the rate of the cells and the body's metabolism functions, including growth and development as well as the body's temperature.

Hyperthyroidism can be described as a medical condition which causes the thyroid gland to release excessive amounts of thyroid hormones. It's caused by thyroid nodules that are too active or the occurrence of a disease known as Graves disease.' Graves disease is more prevalent among women aged 40 or less. It is characterized by anxiety eye puffiness, low or high temp, weight gain and hand shakes. The doctors often prescribed medications for hyperthyroidism and radioactive iodine in order to decrease TSH production.

Hypothyroidism can be described as a medical condition that causes the thyroid gland to produce lower levels of hormones. The most common among women over the age of. It can alter all aspects of metabolism including the body temperature, heart rate and digestion systems.

The most common symptoms of hypothyroidism are constipation, weight gain, fatigue, and dry skin.

Hypothyroidism diagnosis that is accurate and safe and treatment are offered in hospitals. Treatment using synthetic thyroid hormones is extremely efficient.

21st century lifestyles causing chronic stress

The world health organisation has stated that stress is the 21st century health Epidemic. Certain life events, such as being married and the birth of your child divorce, the loss of the love of your life and financial struggles, as well as bankruptcy cause a feeling of normal tension that lasts longer than anticipated.

The multitude of worries in life cause stress. You fret about your partner's finances, money families, jobs, and even your career. It is also stressful due to perceived threats like mass shootings kidnappings, political anxieties as well as exposure to diseases that are viral or fearing that something bad could occur to you or your family members.

Stress at work is an issue for the beggar today, when compared to the past. Gina Soleil, a workplace mindfulness coach, documents attempts by companies to manage stress from work "In in the 90s the term "work-life balance was coined to refer to the ability to manage everything and do it without stress".

The emphasis was on setting priorities through proper time management. The middle class enjoys the possibility of balancing their health, career and social lives. But, many people were entangled with more responsibilities and tasks instead of finding that well-deserved equilibrium.

Smart-hard-work was the name of a phrase that was that was coined in the early 2000s as an approach to business that could help the new generation of millennials to meet and exceeding their goals around the clock.

Smart hard work was the name coined in the context of Corporate Americas' response to an engaged work environment and measuring performance on results , not the amount of time in office that is based on the Result only Work Environment (ROWE) concept.

Instead of finding balance employees are taking on more responsibility , resulting in greater stress levels despite their the fact that they have a lot of talent, are hardworking and their only work motivation.

The next decade was ushered into existence with a new slogan, "do more with less." This phrase was coined in the height of the recession in 2008-2009, when more than 8 million jobs eliminated. People who were employed following the recession were given more responsibility to ensure business continuity, and sometimes, they take on more than one job to make up for their declining earnings. Stress at work reached its highest point in the last few decades.

Technology advancements have brought modern, high-end electronic devices like smart devices, apps and sophisticated enterprise applications that promise savings in costs efficiency, productivity and work-life harmony. But, workplace stress is growing, costing corporations in America over $300 billion each year.

A life-long addiction to mobile devices and the need to develop connections with business and personal contacts through social media can affect mental health due to the immense stress load.

Gradually, stress has snuck into the homes of many people and homes, but it's not noticed. Technology has dominated people's lives, causing the need to increase their social media followers, feeling at their beautiful, well-lit photos and lifestyles.

Follow trending hashtags to stay up-to-date on Twitter and crashing live streaming. Responding to texts and WhatsApp messages, and the fear of being missing out on social and family activities.

This activity can create the possibility of disruptions and interruptions in social interaction, as well as bad sleeping habits, which can lead to depression and anxiety.

21st century stressors

A thorough understanding of the real cause of the stress is crucial in removing or managing it. I refer to this as stress diagnosis. It is the deliberate attempt to discover the reasons why the adrenal gland keeps producing cortisol in a constant manner, which puts you on alert, even when asleep.

I briefly discussed a few stressors in the previous part. I will review the seven principal types that stressors fall under in the following chapter.

Stress in life is caused by your responses and actions to events or situations like marriage or facing financial difficulties, as well as objectives. The cause of bankruptcy is a company's failure to meet its obligations; beginning and running a business and possibly expecting your first baby is a traumatic event that makes people insane.

The second category of stressors comes from fears about the potential threats that could be posed by our environment. Fearing mass shootings, the fear of a decline in prices because of climate change crises, political turmoil, and viral infection. These aren't real, but merely a fantasy. In extreme situations it could cause panic attacks.

The third type of stressors is the stress resulting from to unexpected and real-life events. Natural disasters are the reason for being homeless has been associated with chronic disease, loss of job, and even a plane crashes. These unplanned events alter the perspective of people on life shifting from opposition to understanding, and expressions of grief because of these circumstances.

The fourth category of stressors is the direct result of work or life-related activities. Certain occupations are naturally difficult. Some jobs require constant communication for 5 hours a day like customer service. The sport of athletics can be an extremely stressful occupation. Stress at work can also be a the result of having to meet deadlines.

The fifth stressor is psychological. Addiction is a reaction not only to unhealthy lifestyles like drinking and smoking, but also to technological devices like smartphones or social media. Addiction can have a negative effect on mental health and in some instances, can cause social isolation.

The stress of aging can also be psychological. The midlife crisis is the result of aging, leading to an existence-threatening crisis. As people age typically around 40, they start to inquire about everything. They feel agitated as if their lives are ending right before their own eyes. Menopausal changes and the effects of menopausal changes can cause anxiety and doubt. Nora Ephron famously said, "you will not be a permanent, unchangeable you for the rest of your life." This time of apparent biological changes, accompanied by denial and long-term doubts often result in regular mode changes(depression) because of increased body awareness resulting from anger and anger.

The stress-related issues are triggered by social interactions. Blind dates or a seminar and meeting new people online or offline, all of it is caused by our relationships.

The final category of stressors are what I called spiritual stressors. It is a physical manifestation with spiritual implications. It's a result of our relationships with others. The desire to get revenge, the holding of grudges, and the inability accept the actions of people who have offended you result in building the profile of people and their offence and your plan of revenge.

In extreme instances individuals are enslaved to their own burdenswhich is a burden of frustration and rage. The pressure becomes chronic when there is no one to talk about their feelings.

When a disagreement or misunderstanding is triggered, our relationship, it becomes the burden. It is best to speak to older people about it and the stress level decrease dramatically. In the majority of cases, if it goes untreated, it can result in a religious commitment that is too burdensome to bear.

Stress and aging

It is crucial to bring your attention to the unique health condition in our times, known as a midlife crisis - the result of stress that is extreme that has various symptoms for both genders.

The phrase was invented in the year 1957 through Elliot Jacque, a physician and psychoanalyst. He used the phrase in a paper that he gave at a conference with the British psychoanalytical society.

He explainedthat "until now, the world has appeared to be an upward slope without a distant horizon visible. In the last few minutes, I feel to have reached the top of the hill and in front of me is the slope that is downwards with the final destination visible in sight"-far enough away that is it true, however, there is a death-like presence near the end.

He also explained that there is a sexual awakening, promiscuity an inability to appreciate life, hypochondriacal issues over appearance and health, and an obsession with staying youthful.

The time period is full of numerous stressors due to what I call "halfway performance review" with a life-threatening incident.

The Dr. Schwartz, a certified psychoanalyst explained the situation as "many older people are evaluating their lives at work along with their accomplishments, financial health and to which they've reached their targets or goals." A feeling of complete failure for those who feel they had not made any significant progress or those who had a difficult time completing with the job they have chosen, not due to their passion , but because they had enough money to provide for their families. The question is 'how many years do you think it will take?

The third reason is change in the body's biology. As a result of ageing, both genders began to notice the inevitable physical changes that occur in their bodies. Women may experience depression because of their appearance diminishing.

The condition may be caused through a drastic reduction in salary or job loss, or any other event that puts an increase in the burden on men's financial situation, especially when there's a new baby, regardless of whether the kids are older. Men may be tempted to reconsider their choice of spouse, career or previous relationships, their past decisions, or anything else that could be considered that is questionable.

These distinct conditions for both genders that result from numerous stressors could directly impact their health, particularly depression and anxiety.

Diagnostic of Addison Disease Natural Treatment for Addison Disease

The adrenal gland makes two different hormones that are essential for the metabolism of sexual activity and the stress hormone(Cortisol). Adrenal disorder refers to a situation in which the adrenal gland is producing excessive or insufficient hormone.

Addison disease is a medical condition which causes the adrenal glands to release lower levels of hormones as a result of damages in the adrenal Cortex. As per the Dr. George T. Griffins Endocrinologist "the inability to treat the disease generally occurs when 90% or more of the adrenal cortices in both of them are malfunctioning or degraded. "

Adrenal insufficiency may be difficult to recognize in its early stage. Thus, medical professionals typically examine medical history and signs.

Adrenocorticotropic (ACTH) Test for hormone stimulation is commonly used to identify Addison disease. The procedure involves an intravenous injection with an artificial ACTH. A blood sample is taken prior to the injection, and 30 to 60 minutes after the injection. The best goal is to see an increase in the blood cortisol levels. If a test is positive the adrenal gland might cause damage and not be able to respond with this ACTH test. Thus, those with Addison illness will see minimal or no rise of cortisol levels.

The ACTH test might not be accurate for individuals who have experienced secondary adrenal insufficiency that lasted for just a short period of time, since their adrenal gland might not be damaged as it still responds to ACTH.

The Corticotropin-releasing hormone (CRH) stimulation test is another option to identify secondary adrenal fatigue insufficiency. Particularly in situations where it is apparent that the ACTH test isn't easy to do. It's a second-line, non-invasive dynamic test that allows for the precise detection of diseases. An under-average increase in ACTH and possibly 20% increase in cortisol concentrations from baseline indicates pituitary glands as the reason for adrenal insufficiency.

The doctor may perform the test of insulin resistance in the event that the doctor suspects there's a pituitary gland problem or when the test for insulin tolerance isn't as clear. It's the gold standard for getting access to ACTH in addition to the Cortisol Reserve. Injecting insulin into veins followed by the measuring of blood glucose levels at regular intervals.

Imaging and blood tests can be performed to determine the root reason for adrenal insufficiency after being diagnosed as adrenal. This test can determine if tuberculosis is the cause.

Treatment for Addison disease

The treatment for Addison disease involves hormone replacement therapy to regulate the levels of steroids hormones your body isn't making as suggested by your physician.

It is also recommended to take a look at the Mayo Clinic also recommends a little bit to salt(sodium) within your daily diet especially when you exercise hard during hot weather.

Addison disease is only medical issue and I would suggest you to consult your physician.

Test and natural cure for Adrenal Fatigue

There isn't a medically-acceptable screening test to determine adrenal fatigue since it's not a medical issue; rather it describes a set of signs and symptoms that indicate how the body reacts to stress.

The treatment of adrenal fatigue is as important treatment for chronic stress. It is distinct from Addison disease in that the former is a disorder, while it is actually a medical issue.

Adrenal glands can be exhausted in a situation where different medical diagnoses fail to identify Addison or Cushing disease, but the symptoms are obvious.

If, however, you require more information or you're not sure if your symptoms are the result of stress over time or other stress-related issues, there's an assessment kit that you can buy either online or offline to check for adrenal deficiency. It's a self-test kit.

It's called the saliva test for cortisol/DHEAS. It measures the level of the stress hormones cortisol and dehydroepiandrosterone (sex hormones) in your saliva and provides an analysis of how this hormone varies throughout the day. The test kits are provided with do you can do it yourself instructions. Labs like Genova and ZRT allow patients to purchase the test kits on their own.

The most important thing is to speak to an experienced health professional about your concerns and ask whether the test is useful for you. Plan B Medicare includes the test of saliva. It is the World Health Organization and the National Health Institutes (NHI) are able to recognize the saliva cortisol test with precision.

The test for saliva is a good indicator of the steroids (sex as well as stress hormones) within the body. Similar to blood tests, certain labs are more precise than others.

Researchers from the Medical University of Vienna, Austria verified the accuracy of saliva tests to test for burnout levels. According to them, burnout is a sign of health.

"Our latest data show that those who are at risk of burnout could be identified by one saliva sample at an nearly 100 percent accuracy".

The test can reveal a an imbalance in biochemistry that could be the primary cause of chronic fatigue, stress and depression. It also shows obesity and many other chronic illnesses.

How do you manage chronic stress?

The first step in managing stress is to understand the triggers or stressors that trigger you. Triggers include life events, environmental triggers such as social events, natural forces, and stress-related to our work.

They are permanent and temporary strategies to manage stress. The strategies for managing stress are temporary and include strategies to assist you in managing stress for the short or the immediate time.

A short-term approach to managing stress is a way to address different signs of stress. A headache can be treated with an extended break or taking medication to reduce the discomfort. The treatment for fatigue includes energy boosters and medications to ease the symptoms. People who suffer from early morning fatigue can go to the extent of making salt additions to water each day to help brighten their day.

These are all short-term solutions to deal with stress. This will help take tension away.

A report published on Yahoo lifestyle describes how the world-renowned footballer Christiano Ronaldo manages the unique stress from his profession. Ronaldo requires time to take sufficient rest to his ability to perform at a consistent top of his game.

The stress management and sleep experts advise him to get five-times, ninety minutes sleep each night. He also eats at least five times his balanced diet each day.

Jack Dozie of Twitter also does a bizarre thing in managing his stress , which comes from stress that comes with his position. Jack is a regular participant in an ice bath at minimum every day. He fasts on a regular basis.

Traditional stressors and the modern lifestyle cause the stress epidemic that has an enormous impact on the mental well-being.

Unplanned life events such as the loss of a loved one, loss of employment or divorce, chronic illness and serious illness that results due to an accident can result in stress throughout your life.

The necessity to achieve set objectives in the workplace and deal with layoffs if they are not met goals could cause stress in the workplace. Executives in the top ranks and C-executives are able to enjoy the luxury of employing a professional stress management specialist. Others classes of employees might not have the luxury of hiring a stress management expert.

Although A-list stars such as Ronaldo could employ an individual stress specialist who would create a customized stress management program for him, people who aren't celebrities could not afford the expense.

Although it is impossible to avoid stress in the present age, it is also possible to control chronic stress.

There's a shortas well as a long-term method of managing stress. The short-term strategy is aimed to reduce the tendency to fight by keeping the body in control. The long-term strategy will assist to treat the stress hormones.

Short-term strategies for stress management

An acute stress reaction is body's response to an perceived threat. The body's response to stress is immediate and exciting. Examples of these responses include the body's heat, narrowly avoiding accidents on the road, going to an interview for a job or your first meeting.

A single incident of stress should not cause harm. But, a posture that is prone to multiple stressors can affect mental health like panic attacks. It may cause digestive issues and heart attacks, as well as headaches that are acute and other physical health problems.

There are strategies you can employ for managing stress that are acute. For instance, in an interview or a job test when you begin to notice aspects of fear or panic then you should simply breathe deeply and slowly breathe in, breathe deeply, hold your breath and then exhale. Repeat the process as many times as you like. You'll notice that the anxiety and fear disappear. You will feel more relaxed and relaxed.

A remarkable thing happened during that exercise. When you breathe out and in you block this flight-related response. When you breathe deeply and control your reaction, gradually taking control and bring the abnormal response to a stop.

Different strategies are applied to different stressors over the short-term to manage the fight, flight or freeze response based on the specific situation.

Attaining coherence by using 4 by 4 for 4.

I discussed how to control anxiety by breathing. It is essential to comprehend the mechanisms that take place as you deliberate your breathing to make sure you're breathing in a consistent manner.

If we choose to deliberately change our breathing patterns facing panic or fear it stops the involuntary stress response , and create a more balanced balance in our autonomic nervous system.

The autonomous nervous system consists of the natural accelerator (the sympathetic) and decelerator(parasympathetic). When these two essential components that comprise the autonomic nervous system get deliberately activated, we achieve coherence.

At the point of maximum coherence, we can achieve concentration, mental clarity and concentration. Thus, the goal in the short-term is to improve stability in our emotions and improve connectivity to prefrontal cortex.

Stress and anxiety that cause anxiety occurred as the natural accelerator outpaced your natural accelerator. This is why it's vital to control your breathing.

Inhaling deeply your heart rate rises but it slows down when you exhale. Inhaling and exhaling signals are transmitted to the brain, which controls the autonomous nervous system.

Four by four for 4 is the breathing strategy to use when confronted with an overwhelming task that causes anxiety and fear. It's a simple breathing method to turn off anxiety and prepare your body to relax.

Breathe in for four seconds, exhale for 4 seconds, then repeat the process for four minutes.

This process is able to be continued for at least four minutes , until you achieve clarity and coherence. If you're not in the position of having four minutes to go through the process three or seven times will suffice. Sometimes, you won't even be able to keep track of the duration. All you have to do is repeat the process until you reach a level of coherence.

This method will allow you to break the endless cortisol and adrenaline flow that can push you to the edge.

Utilizing the Magical and powerful aromatic qualities of essential oils and scents

The advent of Aromachology has led to a new business based on the psychology of scent. Aromachologist replicate scents. For example, if experienced a sense of relaxation during shopping, the scent that you are experiencing in that moment could be recreated to create the same feeling when other people are shopping.

The study of Aromachology is the effect of various scents on the human mind. The most well-known scent expert Ben Janousek revealed to mail online that by studying the process of Aromachology you can observe how different scents affect the brain.

You might not realize the essential role of smell. It's not just about making you feel happy, but scent can also help you relax your nose when you're feeling exhausted or stressed. Scent can make you feel more relaxed and energetic.

The Aromachologist utilizes a scientific method to study the psychological effects of both synthetic and natural scents on the way we behave and our mood. Aromatherapists aren't as than a holistic medical professional who are based on science.

The Aromatherapist is a proponent of using natural fragrances like essential oils. The Aromachologist recommends the use of both natural and synthetic medicines.

If you are using artificial or natural fragrances it is important to understand that the scents you wear may help you reduce stress for the short-term.

The smell released by scents affects the hypothalamus (the brain's part) which regulates the hormonal system).

The study, published in the journal Advanced Nursing revealed that lavender could help patients in intensive care be less stressed and more optimistic. Jane Ehrman, an integrative and lifestyle medicine specialist said that "you can make aromas that act as a to help you relax in your kitchen , and give the mood that you want when trying to relax."

It is crucial to know that essential oil, with all its magic power is not controlled by the federal government. Therefore, you must review the leaflet for the product prior to making use of it. Skin's reaction to synthetic fragrances can be heightened and it's essential to customize your fragrances as different people react differently to scents.

Essential oils can be used at home to relax after a tiring day and sleep comfortably. Use essential oil in an infuser which fills an atmosphere that is fragrant.

Lauren Lamagna, the director of product for candles that are scented to make you feel homesick explained that "herbal scents like lavender and Rosemary as well as a refreshing floral scent such as ylang-ylang have been proven to lower cortisol levels, improve peace and decrease stress levels."

Certain essential oils that have been shown to ease stress include Rosemary Lavender, peppermint, lavender as well as ylang-ylang and lemon.

Essential oil diffuses from plants and herbs scents are man-made fragrances that are made from oil, which is natural in nature. Synthetic fragrances are produced using synthetic chemical elements that are not present in nature. It is more durable than a different fragrance. Natural fragrance oil is created by separating naturally-derived scent components from a complex scent. There is no natural element to it. It's just a scent. The ingredients that are natural are rose geraniol, citrus limonene and Vanillin made from Vanilla.

Perfumes and fragrances can relieve stress the way essential oils work. Essential oil is a natural substance fragrances are created in chemical elements in the laboratory. Essential oils or perfumes will help to ease stress. If your body is prone to sensitivities to chemicals, you may want to make use of natural fragrance oils instead of synthetic oils.

Pause or Take a Break

Every person has a goal to reach daily. Stress at work is the most prevalent kind of stress. Stress at work is due to the desire to reach and surpass our goals. Most times we fail to appreciate that work is always present. Even when the goal for the day is met and we're enticed to over-deliver.

The management of stress requires awareness. Everyone has the tipping point. The speed that acute stress transitions to chronic stress causes one to aware of the point where the tolerance begins to become difficult. They will take a step back to avoid a breakdown.

After reaching the threshold those who decide to go on with their lives are afflicted with physical, mental and emotional symptoms that rise as stress levels increase. It is important to have the courage at this point to take the difficult decision to lower the levels of cortisol.

A large portion of people are afraid of taking time off to go on vacation due to the fact that they don't feel like they is able to work during their absence or they feel their work load is too burdensome.

Elizabeth Grace Saunders, a time management coach, has identified two types of vacation-related Stress In Harvard Business Review. "I have observed that pre-vacation stress from work generally be divided into two categories that include completing work prior to you leave or getting absent from work."

Some individuals believe their colleagues might be scathing for taking time off, especially in the face of a huge amount of work to be done at work. If they're not there and something bad could occur. The supervisor might even find that they aren't making much progress on a specific task as they had claimed.

This fear could prevent people from taking a vacation While others may attempt to complete their work prior to departing for vacation. Many may even work even while they are away. The additional workload initially could become an additional burden that causes stress in multiple ways. The psychological impact of having being at work while absent can cause stress.

Making plans prior to your vacation can assist in completing some of the essential tasks prior to your holiday. Collaborating with colleagues who could assume the responsibility when you're away can be beneficial. Inviting the colleague within a week or sooner and describing some of the essential tasks that must be completed during your absence, can be helpful.

It is essential to realize that you cannot be productive when working for hours without taking breaks. Make sure to take a break prior to when you fall down.

A break is essential for mental clarity, better performance and focus, as well as more influence circles.

It is important to be able how to decline certain things , and in a specific circumstance. It can help you! Learn to control your time by taking time off of social networks and the constant streams of information.

Reframing Negative and Unplanned Events to create positive experiences

Chronic stress can be the due to unpleasant or unplanned incidents. Cognitive restructuring and cognitive reframing are tools utilized by psychotherapists to treat depression, relationships, post-traumatic disorders, anxiety and even the condition of Addition.

It is a versatile tool with a variety of possibilities. But the focus here is on how you can utilize this effective tool to benefit yourself without the need for a psychotherapist. The focus is on cognitive reframing as it is a much more accessible tool than cognitive restructuring. But, it can be difficult to reframing without restructuring.

Naturally, the daily routines are full of unplanned events which can result in an increase in adrenaline and cortisol levels. As you drove fast to beat your logging hours at work, it was possible that you ran into an unusually busy road, which could cause you to arrive at work later. Even so, your phone is ringing and reminding you of an upcoming meeting.

Your breathing speed increases as your heart beats faster and you begin to think about ways to inform the person calling you that you may be late due to traffic that is unusual. What do you do to resolve this?

Are you planning to grow wings and fly away from crowd? Or, are you planning to smile for a lateness to get to work, because you don't want the Adrenaline or Cortisol levels?

Cognitive reframing is a technique employed in reorganizing things mentally to lessen stress and encourage calm. If properly utilized the cognitive reframing process can transform the mountain into a manageable obstacle.

Cognitive reframing is a way to reframe the negative day into an unintentionally low point within a life that is uplifting, from the loss of a beloved one to a move into a better life and huge traffic, to an intriguing situation. Cognitive reframing may alter the perception of stressors, thus alleviating a substantial amount of stress prior to taking any action to alter the perception of situations.

Cognitive reframing transforms the negative thought pattern of the pessimists and transforms it into positive thinking patterns of optimistic people, as pessimists are subject to more stress and achieve lower levels of success than those who are optimistic.

In a massive crowd For instance the possibility of examining your opinions on traffic. Do you often connect traffic with a negative or stressful situation? Because many people do. Be as realistic as you can. Yes! It is possible that you arrive at your destination later due to the congestion.

It happens, but it isn't something that happens every day. Wouldn't it be interesting to experience all the fascinating situations that traffic creates? passed the same location for years , but not noticing the unique and beautiful design of the structure surrounding. Does the urban planning organization have a great job at the process or did they do a poor job? Do you think it means that there isn't a plan?

What else can you spot in the crowd? Perhaps a young couple in the same car you used to drive in the past 10 years? What memories do you have of the car?

How can we learn something from traffic flow? Patience? or what? How do the drivers coordinate their own actions?

When you shift the negative experience link into the traffic you are in, your cortisol level and cortisol levels stay the same, even when you're in a circumstance that could boost your adrenaline.

The cognitive reframing tool is a great tool to use in any stressful event. It could be the loss of loved ones as well as war, accidents and everything else you could imagine.

Long-term strategies for stress management

These are lifestyle changes that aid the body in building defense against external aggression.

It is crucial to realize that there isn't a single method of dealing with stress that is suitable for each person. Individual stress management is similar to the prescription for a medicine that won't be identical for every person. It's not right to follow the prescription of somebody else since each medicine is dependent on the specific diagnosis and signs and symptoms of each person.

Every person should be aware of the causes of stress. Create a personal or individual plan to address the root causes of stress.

Have you been dedicated to managing stress over the long-term requires gradual changes to your lifestyle. It takes discipline and tenacity to establish a life style that can help you deal with stress effectively.

Joining your Tribe

A reliable social community of family and friends will help you manage numerous stressors in your life. A trustworthy network needs to be substantial. It is important to have a trusted friend who doesn't have an inclination to be sympathetic while listening to your.

An emotional support system offers vital protection during life difficulties. According to the APS Stress in 2015 America survey, the median stress level for people with a supportive system that is dynamic was 5 out of 10, and 6.3 on an scale from 1-10, where 1 is the lowest Stress and 10 is the highest stress.

You may not need a vast network of friends/family/neighbors and colleagues to navigate the negative effect of stress. You will have a small number of people to go to for support. The person with whom you're able to get advice with might be different from others who can offer advice on the subject of your child. Other people could be able to help you deal with the specific tension.

The goal is to lower the stress levels. This means that you have to be careful and deliberate about the selection of your support system. Beware of people who are always negative and critical. Avoid people who rely on alcohol or drugs to deal with stress. They can derail your efforts.

It is important to make time to nurture your relationship and master the art of social interaction to build more connections. Additionally, you require emotional intelligence to know the aspects of your relationship that are worth nurturing.

A way to determine whom to confide in the stress you feel is by identifying people who have succeeded in particular areas. Stress in the marriage could be shared with someone who has a happy marriage. Stress in the workplace is a common issue for people who has a career that is successful. Of course, one should not be critical and critical.

You'll need someone with a specific ability to listen, someone who can show compassion and take on burdens.

Your family is your best option to address personal problems Mother, father or a calm family member with a tendency to listen. For anxiety or stress that needs therapy, professional are preferred.

A member of your family is likely to hug you frequently when compared to the other members of your circle. Cuddle hormones, also known as Oxytocin is a substance produced by the body in response to a the hug or when it touches. Oxytocin can be associated with satisfaction and lower stress. The more hugs you have the greater the amount of Oxytocin levels, and the less stress.

The findings of the 2018 study from researchers at Arizona State University, namely Murphy MLM, Janicki Deverts and Cohen of 404 people who were interviewed each night for two hours. Both studies found that hugging can be linked to a reduction in conflicts, particularly when respondents are having an extremely stressful or conflict-filled day.

The most effective way to expand your circle of friends is to become the solution yourself. You can be a volunteer to do something you're enthusiastic about. The benefit of volunteer work is the fact that you encounter people who share similar interests. They will be willing to take on the burden of you and not judge or be criticizing?

It is important to select to make a decision carefully. Develop the art of listening. Pay attention to the needs of people and show empathy even if you don't know an answer. The act of doing this alone will be alleviating your stress.

Strengthen your mental stamina by meditative mindfulness

It is a hell week. Hell Week is five days and nights of basic conditioning with the maximum of four hours of sleeping hours. Achieving this level of training is both required and sufficient to be able to qualify you to be an Navy Seal.

It's the most demanding week in one of the toughest training programs of the

Military. The trainees are subject to continuous evolution in their training. Every trainee who is evolving carry the Inflatable Rubber Zodiacs boat on their heads, has a timed running and endurance training, crawling through the water, and another demanding underwater exercise.

In the Hell Week test the potential Seal physical and mental strength. The trainees push themselves to the brink. The highest percentage of trainees quit at this point. Naturally, some trainees will think why this training? Why?

Seals have been trained by the Navy to manage operations on any terrain. They are trained to conduct operations in any terrain. Hell Week determines who is resilient and capable of performing operations in nearly all terrains.

It's not always the athletically and physically strong student who wins, but the mentally strongest trainee is the one who excels. In the beginning, the program is designed to accommodate those who have average athletic capabilities.

Mister Webb, a formal Navy deal trainee, explains in his memoir, entitled the "Red Circle" that the Seal's program is intended for the average athletic male to get through.

Webb explained that the test for training is your mental power. It's designed to test you until you're able to handle any job regardless of the challenges.

You might be thinking like: I'm not planning to become the Navy Seal, Delta force, Sas special forces. What does this have to do with me?

What lessons can civilians take from the recruits who have made it through The Hell Week?

Mindfulness.

In a scenario of multiple stressors, thinking about an endless list of things to be done, past events, and the uncertainties/possibilities of the future could drive someone crazy or even incapacitate people from concentrating on the task at hand.

Stress can make you feel depressed and anxious in some instances, and could result in a panic attack.

Mindfulness is the answer!

The deliberate decision to become conscious of the present moment without thinking about the past or looking into the future. It's about staying present in the Now!

Mindfulness to reduce stress and management assists you in coordinating your daily routine to ensure that you don't get overloaded at any moment, no matter what the day.

One bite at time!

If you're faced with a lot of challenges that can make you want to quit, Heroes of the hell week encourages you to break the work into the simple format. Bite by bit.

You can split your whole calendar into month. Divide the week into weeks. Divide the days into weeks and the days into minutes and hours. This is the most important job. The majority of successful men employ this method using.

You know exactly what you'll be doing at each moment. You know where you are and what you want to accomplish each moment and every hour. You'll be aware of when you're your path is not in the plan. They will be able to measure your day. Find the variance and calculate the difference from the overall picture.

The people who became Seals Seal were able to focus on their task for the entire week, without having to deal with thoughts of the task they had completed and anxieties regarding the next task.

Make a plan to live your life one day with a purpose without becoming too self-critical and critical. You can complete your tasks without rushing or feeling stressed.

Mindfulness as a stress-management tool is often criticized by a variety of stressors. For instance, people who have their finances getting sloppy can be apprehensive about mindfulness through segmentation, which breaks up the answer to financial problems into bites. They're now focused in what to accomplish at any given moment and not focusing on mistakes of the past or worrying about the burden that is to come in the future.

Mindfulness isn't simply another type of planning. It's about focusing on the present without passing judgement on the past or worrying over the future.

The art of mastering the Aerobic Fitness program using Autoregulation

A rise in Adrenal as well as Cortisol (mental tension) can have physical effects. The physical symptoms of anxiety can cause additional stress on the mind. Blood pressure is high, resulting in an intense heart beat. Exhaustion and muscle tension. The digestive issue as well as body aches and discomfort. Headaches dizziness, headaches, and sleep disturbance.

The psychological strain of stress is anxiety, insanity, restlessness, insomnia as well as sadness and anger.

Exercises that are fitness-related decrease Adrenaline as well as Cortisol levels. They stimulate production of the hormone endorphins that is essential for mode elevation. The elevated endorphin can trigger positive emotions and euphoria that are essential for an energizing outlook on life. Endorphins work as an analgesic or seductive agent which reduce the perception of pain.

Yoga is a body-mind practice. A blend of controlled meditation breathing and physical postures. Yoga is a combination of physical and mental discipline that is required to bring harmony to the mind, body and breath. Yoga exercises regulate the adrenal glands as it helps keep the Bowden in a state of relaxation. But, Yoga is best practiced under the guidance of a qualified instructor to prevent adverse side effects.

Swimming is another exercise that can completely alter your mood. It increases the production of endorphins which reduces anxiety and tension, and promotes relaxation and sleep. However, it is recommended to keep swimming moderate and performed under supervision.

Running and walking are other forms of aerobic exercise which reduce stress levels. It has mental and physical components. The physical component involves the intentional steps taken to get away from different stressors and surroundings and enjoy the peace. The cognitive part is the one that allows the ability to think and not be interrupted. Thinking is a mental activity necessary to make good decisions.

The brain is stimulated by running and causes it to release endorphins - the positive feelings that are responsible for feelings of high-energy runners and decrease stress hormones. Running allows you to take a break from all the stressors and constant interruptions brought on by media.

While all kinds of Aerobic exercises can help relieve the adrenal gland from fatigue, the most difficult part is mastery and consistency.

How can you ensure consistency and mastery?

It's already available in the public domain that physical exercise helps reduce stress. But, most people find it difficult to get fit. When people gain weight or suffer from other types of physical changes, it happens within a few months or years of neglect to be serious about fitness programs. However, when they are advised to work out, they are discontented as they have not getting any results.

What can something that has been accumulated over the course of a few months or years disappear in one or two days of physical activity? It's because it's an hour-long workout.

In her research, Edward R. Laskowski is a physician at Mayo Clinic, stated that "longer regular sessions of aerobic exercise does not have any distinct benefit over shorter or more frequent sessions. Even a few minutes, spread across the day can provide cardiovascular benefits, and the accumulation of daily activities can bring the health advantages."

The department of human and health services suggests in its physical guidelines for exercise that adults perform at least 150- 300 minutes of moderate intensity or 75-150 minutes of vigorous intensity aerobic exercise each month.

It is essential to regulate your exercise automatically in order to avoid burning out. You can get better by performing better the previous exercise. If your aim is to be the most rigorous training for each routine burning out will happen without assessing your fitness during each routine.

Learning to practice Autoregulation will allow you adapt your work load during every session of training to suit the capacity of your body at that moment. It is possible that you won't be able to complete an hour or longer time, but you'll be able to avoid burning out. This will guarantee that you stay consistent. Autoregulation allows you to keep your the same level of consistency.

The autoregulation process involves the ability to access your current finesses states and capacity. Did you get the needed amount of sleep? Did you have enough food yesterday? Are your muscles fit?

Review how you perform and then adjust it in real-time. Do you require to rest between intervals? Review your overall performance.

Phase 1 The Brakes

As I've mentioned before the system I described earlier is an approach with two components. It is important to realize that in order to put you on the right path we must put an end to the whirlwind we're currently in and begin moving towards the proper direction. You cannot simply change direction when you're exhausted from adrenal fatigue. You must stop the process. This doesn't mean that you need to stop what you're doing in your daily life. You'll be able to carry on your day in the most normal way feasible. It is logical to assume that most of you won't be able stop every stressor in your life, and neither do you need to. As you'll realize in Phase 2 of the program, stress isn't your enemy , and can actually aid you in your healing process.

Let's take a look at the things you should stay clear of before we dive into the steps you can take to completely slow down the adrenal fatigue.

Caffeine

Priorities first. You must reduce your intake of caffeine. There is no need to eliminate it completely from your daily routine however, you should to limit your intake to one cup every day. Caffeine can increase cortisol levels, and is particularly beneficial to people who are experiencing stress in their minds. If you are able, go for green tea that contains polyphenols that can benefit your body and mind. If you cannot resist the lure of coffee after having the first cup of strong coffee opt for decaffeinated coffee to complete your day.

If you think there's a an option to make it through the day without taking one additional shot of caffeine I'm here with the information to assure that it is possible to follow the steps we've provided for you. This is what I've witnessed. that.

Alcohol

Another one that is difficult. Maybe the alcohol makes you feel more relaxed in the evening. I'm not here to argue or teach you about the effects of alcohol consumption. Only you can tell if it's properly used. Alcohol shouldn't be consumed all the time and should not be used to boost your mood. The cortisol levels are increased by alcohol and should be utilized in moderate quantities. Drinking regularly can have negative consequences for your cortisol levels. This means you ought to seriously think about reviewing your drinking practices. If you're unable to temporarily get rid of alcohol you can try drinking half the amount you usually drink. This can greatly help.

Sugar

Do you know that sugar triggers cortisol to release into the body? It's not about sugars found in fruits. Don't confuse them. The Creator of Life put the fruits and vegetable on our planet for us to consume to nourish our bodies and make us healthier and healthy and strong. The body doesn't breakdown sugar in vegetables and fruits like it does when factory-made sugars that are concentrated and absorbed. If something has been sugar-sweetened, or contains an intense sweetener, no whatever the organic nature of it and how natural it is, it can affect your body negatively if are suffering from an immune deficiency condition. If you consume 12 bananas, even though there is a possibility of cramps in your stomach but you're not likely to overstress your cortisol similarly. If you're a diabetic however, this will increase the level of your blood sugar and make you require additional insulin.

The moral is that you'll have to reduce the amount of added sugar. Always eat fruit and veggies, but pay attention during this time on eliminating any form of sweetener. This includes xylitol and stevia. If you aren't able to eliminate it entirely, you can follow the 50% rule and cut the amount you use to half.

Okay, you're aware of what not to do in the first phase of putting the stop to your fatigued adrenals, however let's move on to the ways you can actually end the cortisol imbalance and return you to the level your body is supposed to be.

The most crucial step is to drink a drink that you drink each in the morning to get your adrenals back on track.

Rhodiola, Rooibos and Honey

Honey is a well-known ingredient. is, but with rhodiola and rooibos it is a remedy that is so potent that it could end your adrenal fatigue virtually all by itself. If you only take one step from this book, it is the one that will ultimately stop the fatigue of your adrenal glands from happening. Why?

Let's begin with Rhodiola. Rhodiola (rhodiola rosea) occurs naturally in wild areas of the arctic. It is regarded as to be an adaptogen under ayurvedic terms, meaning that it assists in stabilizing bodily functions of the body. This is known as homeostasis, and it counteracts the effects of stress.

The usage for this plant was discovered inside the Greek work De Materia Medica which was written between 50 and 70 CE by the Greek physician from the Roman army. It is one of the longest-lasting books on natural history in the past.

In Russia Rhodiola has been utilized for many years to aid those who deal with the cold weather and stress in daily life. In traditional Chinese medicine, it's called hong jing tian . It is utilized to treat temporary relief from the symptoms of stress, such as the weakness and fatigue.

Rhodiola has been found to ease stress, combat fatigue, ease signs of depression (although it is not completely) and improve the function of the brain and assist in controlling the symptoms of type 2 diabetes. Additionally, it has beneficial effects on the bedroom. Rhodiola has been proven to improve sexual pleasure, pleasure sexual pleasure, and the reaction to gasps.

There are certain guidelines that you should follow in order to maximize the benefits the benefits of this herb. The most crucial is to never use it before going to bed. The adaptogen isn't designed to be employed as a sleeping aid. It won't make you sleepy. The ideal and best timing to take it is in the morning as it helps regulate your cortisol levels that should be elevated in the morning. It will also will give you an energy an energy boost before you start your day. It's not a stimulant, however it is recommended to begin by taking a portion of the recommended dose over the first couple of days. The best method for getting Rhodiola is to take an tincture that comes in the form of liquid, instead of pills. It is faster into your body, allowing it to get your journey in the right direction.

Don't do this more than two times during the course of the day. The second time should be right after lunch or just prior to the time the typical afternoon slump that makes it feels like you want to take an afternoon nap. You don't want your cortisol to drop here, we'd like to remain in a healthy state so that when dinner is served and the time for bed rolls in, the cortisol levels are declining instead of rebounding.

The maximum dose of the tincture would be 1 tablespoon, twice daily.

If you wish to get more benefits from Rhodiola, it is recommended to mix it with tea rooibos. Rooibos tea is a plant which grows within South Africa. It is often referred to as bush tea or redbush. Locals would climb up steep mountain slopes to preserve the leaves, and then beat them on the flat rocks to activate their healing properties.

Rooibos tea is free of caffeine, and loaded with antioxidants that can help fight stress. The problem of Rooibos can be that antioxidants present in your blood have a short lifespan and don't work for long. It is necessary to drink the tea throughout the day. When it is combined with rhodiola, it creates a synergistic impact that allows quercetin and the luteolin to be absorbed by the body for longer. Both antioxidants are proven to kill cancerous cells in tests in the lab. Additionally, rooibos is also an effective bronchodilator. If you are suffering from respiratory issues, it may aid in reducing resistance to the respiratory system and increase the flow of air. It works similarly on blood vessels by relaxing them, helping in lowering blood pressure as well as blood flow to reproductive organs.

Mix in honey and you'll have the trifector powerhouse. Honey is another of the natural healers of nature. Honey is a great source of antioxidants. They can help lower blood pressure, reduce cholesterol levels, and lower the triglycerides level and have an impact on your heart. Honey is also high in B vitamins, which are essential for the production of testosterone. Readers Digest names it as one of their top 20 aphrodisiacs.

Honey, in our case aids in lowering cortisol although only slightly which is good. We don't wish to get rid of cortisol, and neither will you. We are trying to control it. When you mix it with the other ingredients it will give you an adrenal fatigue remedy that, after several days, will bring back that energy to take on the world. However, do not ignore it. This doesn't mean you have to go back to how you were prior to. It is important to finish phase 1 as well as Phase 2. Most people experience an increase in wellbeing, only to return to their old routines. Don't fall into that trap.

Let's see what else is included in Phase 1.

B Vitamins

I cannot emphasize enough how vital B vitamins can be to the overall wellbeing of your health wellbeing. The consumption of B vitamins in a B vitamin combination that contains B1, B2 as well as B5 and B6, B7, and B12 could result in life-changing effects in those who are deficient. Deficiting in B12 alone can trigger a myriad of adverse consequences. If you are often anxious or need to cry too often it's likely you're not getting the adequate dose of

B12. If you're experiencing simple memory issues such as forgetting what you've put in your bag or not remembering names, it may be a B12 problem.

If you are taking the B vitamin combination that contains all of the various B Vitamins, they can aid in these ways:

B1 - Produces neurotransmitters inside the brain. It is beneficial for heart health and prevents hand numbness and tingling.

B2 is vital to produce energy and helps the body breakdown fats. It can help with inflammation, skin problems, and loss of hair.

B3 alters the way that the body utilizes the energy that comes from protein, carbs and fats. It is beneficial for people who drink excessively and suffer from chronic inflammation.

B5 is required by the body to process pantothenic acids to increase energy and speed up metabolism. It can help with anxiety and bad sleep.

B6 plays a part in the enzyme reactions that occur in the body as well as brain development. It is beneficial to those who have an immune system that is weak as well as those suffering from an autoimmune disorder.

B7 - Maybe you've heard of biotin which aids cells in communicating between them. It helps with fatigue and weak nails.

B9 - This is among the most essential ones. It is located in leafy green vegetables however we do not have enough. B9 is vital for cell division, as well as the metabolism of amino acids and vitamins. It helps those who suffer from the symptoms of heart palpitations, weakness headaches, irritability, and heart palpitations.

B12 - Aids in the creation of fresh red blood cells as well as the brain's neurologic function. It helps those who suffer from mental fatigue, memory issues and depression.

There is also evidence that if you take B complex supplements with the rhodiola tea it reduces discomfort in the body. If you feel that you'd rather press the snooze button , and stay asleep for an couple of hours, then use a high-quality B complex.

St. John's Wort OR an Anti-Depressant

The issue isn't uncontroversial and it must be debated. I'm not here to convince you to be on a medication. It is up to you and your physician to decide. This is my attempt to let you know that if you're contemplating taking an antidepressant or you are already on one, that you're not all on your own. It's okay to seek assistance if you require it. If you're struggling with depression or anxiety or other mental health issue that is causing adrenal fatigue, do not feel guilty regarding having a medications. Particularly if you notice that it has helped you in the past.

There are a myriad of adverse effects associated with prescription drugs that is why I'm not going to recommend taking any specific one, if you decide to take it. If you're completely opposed to taking prescription drugs I'm right there with you. I would always argue with my doctor over the benefits of the drugs but that's not something we can debate here. I've used an antidepressant and have found certain benefits, as well as negative side consequences. This is all up to you and your physician to determine depending on your specific situation, but I do not want people who are taking medication to be treated or criticized in any manner.

If you feel frequently anxious or depressed and are not taking any prescription medication like Warfarin or any other medication which affects the serotonin levels similar to SSRI's and antidepressants are, then take a look at St. John's Wort. It is a popular remedy in Germany, St. John's

Wort is more frequently prescribed in the hands of physicians than Prozac and can be purchased at health food stores without prescription. It is crucial to be aware that you should not, under any circumstance blend St. John's Wort with any other medication that alters serotonin levels. Talk to your doctor and look up any medication you take to determine the presence of any contraindications. Input "St. John's Wort" along with the name of your drug to see if any results pop up. The use of two medicines that affect the serotonin levels could result in serotonin-related syndrome that could be fatal, but it's not common.

St. John's Wort has been used as early in 1686 to treat ailments and has been proven to be as effective as SSRI's but with less negative side effects. Be sure to ensure that the product contains at the very least 0.3 percent Hypericin, and follow the directions in the label.

If you want to stay clear of any of these choices You are able to opt out of both.

This is for people who also struggle with anxiety or depression.

Ashwagandha along with Red Reishi

Ashwagandha is another adaptogen which has a long history of medicinal use. It aids in controlling the levels of cortisol and improve the function of your brain. If you notice that you suffer from mental fog and trouble concentrating you'll love the advantages of Ashwagandha. Since around 6000 BC, ashwagandha was used to treat ailments like impermanence, premature aging and emaciation. It also helped to improve sleeping patterns.

Nowadays, the benefits are numerous which include balancing stress levels and its impact upon the nerve system through stimulating the pathways of the brain to produce GABA A neurotransmitter which can help maintain calm and the muscle tone. Ashwagandha can be helpful in stimulating the reproductive system of females and males, it can help with joint pain, the health and immune system, and overall health. If taken in the morning or just before bed can aid in balancing your cortisol and, over approximately two weeks, it will help you to get a great night's rest. Some find that the results occur much faster than this.

If ever there was an adaptogen that could be used alongside Ashwagandha, it's red Reishi. This is a mushroom that has been utilized extensively by those experiencing fatigue. Particularly for those recuperating from cancer. Red reishi improves the immune system, lowers your stress reaction, boosts sleep and can even provide the ability to heal your liver. Although it's an actual mushroom, it combats candida overgrowth , and also supports equilibrium.

It is of paramount importance, however, when you take supplements, you do your research and find the dosage that is appropriate for you. I suggest adhering to the amount recommended on the bottle, and then increasing the dosage by 50% or more at the most.

Be cautious not to take multiple supplements at the same time. It's okay to take the supplements we've compiled however, if you're already taking other supplements, think about adding them to your regimen so that they're taken as a whole. It's difficult for kidneys and your liver to constantly be bombarded by supplements. They can result in organ failure when they are taken frequently. The body shouldn't require a plethora of supplements in order to heal itself in the short amount of time herbal supplements and supplements can be very beneficial.

Acupressure Mat

If you've not had the opportunity to use an acupressure mat and you're not taking advantage of a fairly affordable method to stimulate meridians within your body. It's like Acupuncture. Acupressure mats can be bought from Amazon or at an acupuncture shop for around $30. It's a mat made of hundreds of spikes made of plastic that are sticking through it. Doesn't that sound nice? If you lie down on it and lie down, it releases endorphins that are like opioids. Endorphins are your body's painkillers and can induce the sensation of euphoria.

It forces you to concentrate on the present as well as the moment in which you are. With the spikes piercing the skin, it's tough initially to think of other things. After a couple of minutes, the pain will ease and the circulation of your body begins to improve. A lot of people find that lying on the mat prior to going to they go to bed helps them relax as well as helps to prepare their body to sleeping.

Delayed Graduation

If, as we said earlier, you're suffering due to adrenal fatigue you might have begun to seek out ways to make you feel better even if it's only for short bursts. We've observed that people suffering from adrenal fatigue take impulsive decisions in search of satisfaction and joy. This can be seen from unhealthy habits like drinking in a binge or at evening, daily use of drugs and shopping online every day, going through your social media several times throughout the day, eating out frequently or heavy consumption of pornography and staying up late to check your phone and much more.

The body begins craving dopamine stimulants to help you get through the difficulties you're experiencing. However, the dopamine begins to wear off in such a short time that you don't feel content. It is a good opportunity to evaluate your routines and habits and take note of those that stand out as a dopamine rush or immediate gratification.

The issue is, what could I do to modify my desire for gratification? That's where the work begins. Recognizing the areas of your daily life that give you a quick rush in pleasure can be the initial step however replacing those short hit with more lasting actions will yield dramatic results.

The best method to accomplish this is to study. Visit your local bookshop and browse through the self-help section and locate an self-help guide that is suitable for your needs. There are a lot of books which can benefit you. In the next phase, you should set a goal for reading 10 to 15 pages each day. A mere 10 pages a day is equivalent to 300 pages per month or even a book every month. Simply by adding this routine to your daily schedule you will be filled with motivation and passion that can have life-changing outcomes.

There are numerous activities you can choose to do to defer your pleasure. Exercise, yoga, walking writing, cooking knitting or having a chat with your friends are all positive ways to boost serotonin levels, which will increase your happiness. One thing that appears to offer the most significant benefit , aside from spending time with your loved ones is cleaning. The research has proven that cleaning your house or a specific space or room at your workplace or in your home and thoroughly cleaning it can have a huge impact on your health and well-being as well as the reward centers of your brain.

It's usually evident when you see someone suffering from instant gratification by simply entering their home or in their car or at work. People who are hung up on instant gratification as well as dopamine rushes tend to shy away from bigger tasks such as cleaning. It's astonishing the amount of times this occurs and it's not only people that are lazy. From the wealthy to the poor, the majority of people struggle with keeping their homes clean without hiring a professional. The majority of us dismiss it as the fact that we don't have enough hours between work and our kids, but it's just not feasible. You could be right. Be aware of your reality is.

Phase 2. THE RESET

Many ask "How long will phase 1 run?" or "How long should I finish Phase 1 before moving on to the phase 2?" and the answer is easy. There isn't a right answer. It is up to you to decide. It could be that you must stick to Phase 1 for a week or keep it going up to 3 months, or longer. You don't need to end Phase 1 before you can move on to Phase 2. Make sure that you're feeling that you're cortisol levels beginning to stabilize.

Sodium Bicarbonate Single Day Cleanse

If you've been under stress for a long time, your body can become extremely acidic. Research has shown that acidic environments aid in the growth of cancer cells to develop. If cortisol is running through our body for too long, acid is built in our bodies. The blood and body must have an acidity approximately 7.35 or 7.45. One method to test the pH of your body is to purchase pH test strips at the neighborhood health foods store and dip them into your saliva in the morning, before you consume food, drink or clean your teeth. These things can alter the pH of your mouth. When you remove the test strip from your mouth, compare it with the instructions that the strips come with. Most people suffering from adrenal fatigue be able to detect a pH below 7.35 and typically in the upper 6's.

One option to aid in resetting our bodies is by doing one day of salt bicarbonate cleansing. Sodium bicarbonate (Baking Soda) has a high pH. Baking soda is already used for baking purposes, which means you're aware that it's safe to consume. We're not talking about anything. To perform this sodium bicarbonate cleansing, you should buy the top product and that is not Arm and Hammer brand, since it contains aluminium in it. You can purchase best baking soda of good quality at your local health food store or the grocery store.

You'll require the four-liter (1 gallon) Jug of distilled water , as well. Distilled water is pure H2O. The reason that we don't drink it as often is that it is able to bond to minerals and toxins within the body, and pull out the waste as. Ideal for the removal of toxins, not so great at removing minerals we require. In a certain way it's extremely useful.

Add 3 teaspoons of sodium bicarbonate to the four-liter (1 gallon) container and shake it. The bicarbonate should fully dissolve . This can take three to four minutes. Your goal is to drink up the entire container of water. It is recommended to stay clear of drinking or eating anything up to dinner time, aside from your baking soda drink.

Through the day, you could notice muscle twitches, that are caused by bicarbonate, which releases C02 in your body. It is also possible to see gas bubbles disappearing from your stomach. Sodium bicarbonate eliminates the air and gas bubbles inside us. If you are suffering from flatulence, this can cleanse you completely and last until the next meal.

It is possible to do this once a month if discover that your pH is too low. Don't do it every day, however, because you need acids in the digestive tract in order to digest the food you eat.

Meditation

I suggest you improve the flow of oxygen through your system. You can achieve this through exercise , or simply taking a 15 minute MINDFUL walk every day. What exactly is an mindful walk? For one hour of walking while your thoughts are in a tense state, or contemplating the various things that are going on in your daily life may not be the same as fifteen minutes of mindful walking.

Mindful walking isn't difficult to master. Simply walk, taking each step with the intention of to heal your body every step ahead. Make sure to breathe deeply and let oxygen enter your lungs as you walk. If you're able, go outside. See the sky in the distance and consider how large of a planet we live on. Imagine the energy of the universe or the earth into your body, and cleansing it. You'll get more energy and health from this 15 minute walk that you wouldn't otherwise. It can also assist you clear your mind, a kind of meditation.

There are many people who talking about their meditation or what you can do to practice meditation. It's not always sitting on your back with seven candles while you sing "Ohm" at yourself over the course of three hours. Meditation involves getting rid of your thoughts, staying present in the moment and focusing on yourself. Avoiding thinking about the future or past. If we dwell on the past too much it can cause us to get stuck. We can also get stuck when we consider the future we're creating. In this instance, you need to concentrate on the here and right now. In the moment that you are. The healing process your body is doing, and the joy for living. The act of gratitude and appreciation can help you heal faster throughout your life. You can also say "I I love your" to yourself when you walk. If you are finding saying you are a good person is difficult I'd recommend to read a good book on the self and forgiving. Both of them could cause your heartache, and add to the feeling of burning out.

Journaling

If you are suffering with adrenal fatigue it is likely that your brain is not functioning at its peak. There could be cognitive fatigue, brain fog and low concentration. If you've experienced immediate gratification, your brain may not be in the best state it could be. There's a way to reset your mind, one that research has shown to be among the most crucial aspects of regaining your positive energy within your life. This is journaling.

It doesn't mean that you must create a little book each day. Also, it doesn't mean you need to divulge all your thoughts and private thoughts in an article, even though you could choose to share your thoughts as it's probably not going to hurt your feelings.

The process of healing journaling is to write one page of paper before going to going to bed every night. It's possible to write more, but one page is all you require to reap the benefits. It is important to note that this should be done manually. There's something that happens in writing your words on paper instead of typing it into the computer. Handwriting is a kind of art. In the past, not everyone was able to write or read and those who could write were usually considered to be artists. Be aware that when you write using your fingers, you're an artist who can create a unique way to put thoughts on paper.

Most importantly, writing with your hands has been proven to be more memorable for you brain than typing. This means that you will be able to remember the notes you made on paper more easily than use your computer or phone.

Your journal should contain the following.

1. A date

2. Two things you are happy about from the day you had

3. One thing you'd like to have done differently

4. The rest of the page in whatever you are thinking about.

Our brains are constantly bombarded with media and information and we don't give them enough the chance to unwind and decompress. We keep filling them with data however we don't give them the chance to organize and re-run especially with regards to our emotions. It's your chance to let whatever thoughts your mind requires to be released and speak to you. It's time to be open to what's happening within yourself, without judgment. Perhaps you're mad at yourself for some thing. Perhaps you're feeling upset about something, but have been pushing the thoughts into the abyssal regions of your mind in the hope to avoid the emotions associated with the thought. Perhaps you're angry over something someone else has done to you or the other person has done to you. These are the opportunities you have to let out your feelings take note of them, be grateful to them and take a step forward. Perhaps you notice that something similar appears on your diary day in and day out telling you that you must work on whatever it is.

Our minds need space to clear out certain things that keep moving around in their. Clear your mind.

Sleep

I'm not going into this topic because it's obvious. It's obvious that you need to get enough sleep to recharge every day. If you're working 2 shifts, and you're barely getting enough sleep and you're not getting enough sleep, so be it. Try to get up in the appropriate time every evening. Do not stare at your phone at night, because the light coming from the device trick your mind into believing it's a daytime and stops melatonin from being a constant presence, making you feel tired in normal situations. Reading before bed has helped a lot of people to fall asleep which is why this might be the perfect time to take in 10 pages.

Stress

The most crucial for the very last. Stress.

Many of us think that stress is the main factor leading to the greatest problems due to the adrenal fatigue we suffer from. But the truth is that we all experience stress. It's unavoidable. Stress itself isn't the problem. Let me repeat that. Stress is not the problem.

It is the reason people are most likely to be upset. They claim, "Stress is 100% my problem. If I didn't feel stressed and less pressure, then I'd feel happier and well."

It's actually the furthest thing from reality. Stress can be beneficial to our bodies, but we don't know whether or it isn't. Stress isn't what is the problem, but how we deal with the stress. This could be the reason for the contradiction. I'm here to inform that stress will forever be part of our lives. Children, work or aging family members and death, money, relationships, world problems and more. It's never ending. It's a constant swarm of negative thoughts. This makes it feel that the burden of all this is too much and we want to get to get rid of it all.

As I've come realize, there's no way to escape this game. However, there are ways to assist you in coping so that you can go through your day with joy and a feeling of achievement. If you have read

The Upside of Stress by Kelly McGonigal or watch her 20-minute TED Talk, you will discover a variety of methods and strategies that can assist you. Imagine a child who is the first to learn how to walk. What advice would you offer to a child who feels that walking is too hard and wish they never had to confront the difficulty of walking? They'd be thrilled with a snack and pee while lying down in front of a TV for the rest of time. You'd tell them that they're insane and be up and go again.

Check yourself. If you're struggling, that's fine. Everybody goes through it. Every person struggles at one point or another. That's the reason why you're doing this reset , and the reason why you're going through this guide. You're looking to be more relaxed. You'd like to be happier and I'm betting you'd be even more happy if could manage your day-to-day stress instead of trying to avoid them.

The process of avoiding stress can be stressful and is the reason for burning out for many. It is essential to make a shift in your mindset and recognize that stressors are bound to keep getting worse, but you're likely to get better at your handling of stressors.

A very effective tools you can employ is the activated switch. When you feel anxiety or stress it activates similar neural circuits that are responsible for excitement. In both situations the heart rate rises and you feel feelings of stomach butterflies, and your cortisol levels begin to increase. There is only one difference: your attitude. If you are feeling stressed and cortisol begin to begin to rise, tell yourself that you're excited. You can manage the tension. Most importantly, assure your body that you're in good hands. Whatever your current stress, it won't keep you from feeling content.

It's not an overnight solution. For many, our minds have been taught to be fearful of stress. This triggers the wrong response within our bodies. It is necessary to change the sequence, so that we are not afraid of stressful events. Most of the time, stressors mean that you are faced with a problem you need to fix or do. One of the most effective ways to boost your general health is by giving back to others and fixing something that somebody else has broken. When you believe in the bigger picture of the work you do it can assist in relieving some of the pressure that stress puts on you.

If you can find ways to reduce stress in your life, you should look at them as well. Don't put all your efforts to eliminating stress because that's not likely, and it's not healthy for you. When we overcome challenges and overcoming obstacles, we are filling up the reward centers in our brains. This allows us to indulge in the sweets we offer ourselves as long as they aren't regular rewards that meet our desires for instant gratification.

Spiritual

No matter what you believe about spirituality You've probably heard the expression "MIND BODY, MINDS, and the

SOUL" and there's an explanation behind it. Our bodies consist of cells and organs, which are managed by our minds , and are connected to the universe through our soul. It is not my intention to force you to believe in any nonsense spiritual diarrhea However, I'm going to give you steps to increase your overall health and well-being. The way you use it is your choice. If you'd like to skip right to the end then, of course, take it. If you're interested in all the information and are able to take a second section that I went through to recover myself be sure to pay attention.

There are three steps you should do to heal throughout your journey, which is connected to your soul. It's not required to believe in the existence of a God or a god, but you should be aware that somewhere out there in the universe there is a chance that there is a source of energy source that powers the stars and the sun. There's no harm in wanting to tap into this energy or higher energy and use it to aid in healing. Even if you're the deepest atheist in the world, and don't believe in a connection with the energy of the universe but there are three things I'd like you to take action on. They're all in a certain order:

1. Make yourself feel good about yourself. Everyday. If you're unable to declare it, or don't believe in it when you speak about it, then you ought to take a stroll in the park, and consider the reasons. It is possible that you're holding feelings of guilt, anger, sadness or any of a variety of other emotions within your body, and these may be holding you back from getting better.

2. Forgive. Forgive people for their mistakes toward you, but most important, accept forgiveness for yourself! We've all made mistakes. We've all made bad choices. We've all taken wrong path at various points throughout our life. There is

no way to alter the past. Take a moment to think about the events that have impacted your life in negative ways. Note them down. Find them. Display them to yourself, after which you can burn them. Use a pencil to cross the lines a hundred times. Remind them that you're no longer regretting them. You've held them all the time. You accept the mistakes you've committed. It's been a while since I've met anyone who's perfectly. Whatever the way you did, you're worthy of gratitude and love.

3. Believe that you're healing. Imagine you in your ideal body that you would like to have. Imagine your body healthy with vitality, energy capable of handling any the stress comes your way. Remind yourself each day that "I am getting better." Sometimes, your body requires a reminder of what you're doing.

Ok, that's that. If you're looking for the time to take some exercise or reflect or write down your negative thoughts you have in your mind to face them with forgiveness and love Do it. Remember that the solution to every problem is love. The most important thing is to love yourself.

Chapter 6: What Is Adrenal Deficiency?

Inadequacy in the adrenal glands is because the organs of the adrenal fail to produce enough cortisol, and, in some cases, aldosterone. The production decreases when your adrenal cortex (the organ's outer layer) is destroyed. This is often the case in the case of an illness of the immune system that causes your body to attack the organs. It could also be caused by cancers as well as tuberculosis, among other types of illnesses. The is often referred to as the essential adrenal deficit.

The adrenal gland that is not functioning properly, which is more common than the normal structure, occurs because you require more the hormone adrenocorticotropin (ACTH) which is the chemical released through the pituitary organ. If your pituitary organ doesn't produce enough ACTH, the adrenal organs aren't producing enough cortisol. Adrenal exhaustion occurs when your adrenal organs aren't able to perform as they should. The diet for adrenal exhaustion is advancing the legitimate value of adrenal organs' supplementation of the circulatory system, and expanded use of solid substances within the body. The body also developed anxiety symptoms.

This diet is similar to the majority of suggested weight loss plans that generally comprise high-protein foods.

Vegetables

Entire grains

The aim is to boost your energy levels regularly so you don't have to take in the supplements you have put away.

The diet to treat adrenal weakness is still being studied. It is largely due to the fact that experts are still examining the possibility of adrenal weakness. It has been proven that having a healthier diet and adopting an improved way of living will help you have an enhanced outlook on life both personally and mentally.

What is Adrenal Exhaustion?

The reason for adrenal fatigue is constant pressure and adrenal inadequacy. The adrenal organs are responsible to produce cortisol. Cortisol is the chemical responsible for managing your pulse. If you're stressed your adrenal organs release cortisol. Cortisol triggers an insusceptible dialed back framework, and also to an adjustment of blood pressure.

If you are experiencing constant stress or anxiety your adrenal organs might not be producing enough cortisol. This is known as adrenal inadequacy. It is a medical issue that can be analyzed. The term "adrenal exhaustion" is not considered to be an analysis of clinical significance. A few experts are aware of the ongoing stress.

Adrenal Insufficiency The Reasons

The term "adrenal weakness" is not a recognized clinical diagnosis. It is a term that refers to a variety of unclear adverse effects, such as body throbs and exhaustion anxiety, rest aggravations and stomach-related issues.

The adrenal glands of your body produce a variety of chemicals that are essential for the rest of your life. The medical term "adrenal deficiency" is a reference to the lack of production of one or more of these substances due to an infection that is not obvious or a medical procedure.

Side effects and signs of adrenal deficiency could include:

*Fatigue

*Body is throbbing

Unexplained reduction in weight

*Low blood pressure

*Lightheadedness

*Loss of hair on the body

Skin staining (hyperpigmentation)

The presence of adrenal deficiency can be assessed through blood tests and incitement tests that reveal low levels of adrenal chemical.

The advocates of the adrenal exhaustion discovery claim that this is a mild form of adrenal deficiency caused through persistent pressure. The most controversial theory for the fatigue of your adrenal glands is that your adrenal organs don't have the capacity to keep up with the demands of constant extreme stress. The blood tests that are currently in use that support this theory, aren't enough sensitive enough to determine small decreases in adrenal function but your body's.

It's confusing to experience adverse effects that your doctor's office can't immediately determine. However, allowing the unnoticed conclusions of an inexperienced doctor could leave the real cause -such as fibromyalgia or melancholy not being discovered, and it causes severe harm.

the Theory behind It

Your body's insusceptible structure responds by firing when you're stressed. The adrenal organs which are the tiny organs located in the kidneys, respond to pressure by releasing hormones like adrenaline and cortisol. These chemicals are crucial to you to have an "instinctive" response. They increase your pulse as well as your pulse. According to the theory in the event you experience long-haul pressure (like the death of a family member or legitimate illness) the adrenal organs get worn out due to the delay in the production of cortisol. This is when adrenal exhaustion starts to take hold.

What are the signs of adrenal issues?

There are a variety of ailments that could cause problems in the adrenal organs' work. Adrenal organs are tiny and are made up of enjoyed triangles. They can be found just above each kidney. They are also known as suprarenal organs. They are responsible for making chemical substances that you need to maintain your digestive system, circulation strain, the resistant system and the stress reaction in equilibrium. Adrenal issues are the result of your organs producing too much or insufficient amounts of certain chemical substances. The adrenal glands release chemicals that comprise hydrocortisone (additionally known as cortisol) as well as adrenaline and aldosterone.

Imagine dominoes and the way that the domino set off an ensuing chain reaction, making the next domino in line fall down. If something happens and the next domino does not take note of the event it is destroyed.

What are normal kinds of Adrenal Problems?

There are a variety of conditions that can be identified in the adrenal organs. Most likely the most well-known are:

Addison's illness, also known as adrenal deficiency. In this condition there is a lack of cortisol, and also aldosterone.

Cushing's condition. When you have this issue your levels of cortisol levels are high. This can happen to large doses of steroids are prescribed to treat certain conditions.

Congenital adrenal hyperplasia. The term refers to a hereditary condition where your adrenal glands don't produce cortisol effectively. Then, ACTH is elevated. Dependent on the deformity, greater amounts of male chemical can be created.

Adrenal organ concealment. It is a form of adrenal deficiency that can be associated with external cortisol wellsprings or engineered chemicals such as prednisone and dexamethasone.

*Hyperaldosteronism. If you suffer from this condition the body produces an excess amount of aldosterone that could cause a rise in pulse and potassium incongruity.

*Virilization. This is a condition that occurs when your body produces lots of male sex chemical and is only evident in females or males who are in their teens prior to pubescence.

There are also conditions of the adrenal organs that have been identified as having changes (growths). They include the growth of the adrenal organs. The growths may disrupt the chemical yield, however they generally are not cancerous.

*Adrenocortical carcinoma. This rare condition is a reference to the formation of diseases in the adrenal organ's exterior layer.

*Pheochromocytoma. If you suffer from this disease your organs produce lots of epinephrine as well as norepinephrine, which can increase your the heart rate or cause it to be a bit faster.

*Pituitary cancers. Unusual growth on the pituitary organ could cause adrenal organ problems by causing an increase in the quantity of chemical produced in the organs of adrenaline. ACTH producing growths can cause Cushing's illness. If the growths are massive, they may cause pressure on pituitary gland and result in an insufficient amount of ACTH and possibly adrenal deficiency.

How Common Are Adrenal Problems?

Adrenal issues can occur to anyone. Within the specific conditions certain conditions may occur more frequently in women than men, for instance, Cushing's syndrome.

Inadequacy of the adrenal glands is a common occurrence when you've been taking the glucocorticoids (like prednisone) for a long period of time, then you cease excessively quickly instead of tightening and reducing gradually. It could also result from of tumors that are present in the pituitary glands, which push on normal pituitary cells as well as from medical procedures or radiation that affects your pituitary gland.

The phases of Adrenal Fatigue

Crisis The meaning of the word might be a bit clearer. The term "adrenal emergency" refers to an health-related crisis. It's the largest complexity of adrenal dysfunction and is triggered due to a severe deficiency of cortisol. An adrenal emergency could be dangerous. Signs of an adrenal emergency are:

Insomnia in the lower part of your body that is rapidly onset. Spouting and running.

*Weakness. The loss of consciousness and confusion.

Low blood glucose

*Low strain on the circulatory system.

If you are suffering from adrenal deficiency it is essential to always have an injectable form of glucocorticoid medicine with you. Additionally, you must wear some sort of medical-grade adornments featuring the information. Be sure that your family members understand how to administer an infusion in the event of a situation. Other chemically irregular characteristics and signs can occur in the context of adrenal disorders. They can be caused by having an excess in potassium (hyperkalemia) or low levels of sodium (hyponatremia) in your blood.

What are the risk factors Concerning Adrenal Issues?

In general, the bases of adrenal disorders aren't identified. However, certain type of adrenal problems are linked to genetic traits. Other conditions may trigger more frequent regularity in the event that you have to take or choose to take certain types of medication, for instance steroids. Steroids are used to treat various diseases, but you need be aware of their numerous side effects.

What is the cause of Adrenal Problems?

Adrenal organ disorders can be caused by problems with the organs themselves that produce excessive or insufficient chemicals. They can also be due to issues with different organs, including that of the pituitary. Genetic factors can also play an impact on certain adrenal disorders. However, it is not clear that anyone is aware of the reason for the issues they cause.

What are the effects of Adrenal Issues?

The signs and symptoms of adrenal disorders change depending on the chemical that are affected. Many of the symptoms of adrenal disorders are similar to symptoms of other conditions.

Effects of inexplicably high levels of cortisone (Cushing's disease) are an increase in body fat with legs and arms are more lean. (A common symptom is referred to as an Buffalo bump refers to an abnormality between the shoulder.)

*Feeling drained and confused.

*The development of hypertension and diabetes.

* Skin that can be smudge-free with no issue.

Wide purplish streak of blemishes across the skin of your stomach.

Signs of high levels of aldosterone are:

www.ingramcontent.com/pod-product-compliance
Lightning Source LLC
Chambersburg PA
CBHW050400120526
44590CB00015B/1758